Clinical Calculations Using Dimensional Analysis

Clinical Calculations Using Dimensional Analysis

Gloria P. Craig, EDS, MSN, RN
Instructor
Iowa Methodist School of Nursing
Des Moines, Iowa

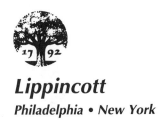

Lippincott
Philadelphia • New York

Acquisitions Editor: Margaret Belcher
Editorial Assistant: Emily Cotlier
Project Editor: Barbara Ryalls
Production Manager: Helen Ewan
Production Coordinator: Nannette Winski
Designer: Doug Smock
Indexer: Lynne Mahan

9   8   7   6   5   4   3   2

Library of Congress Cataloging in Publications Data

Craig, Gloria, 1949–
      Clinical calculations using dimensional analysis / by Gloria
   Craig.
         p.   cm.
      Includes bibliographical references and index.
      ISBN 0-397-55320-X
      1. Pharmaceutical arithmetic.   2. Dimensional analysis.
   3. Nursing—Mathematics.   I. Title.
      [DNLM: 1. Drugs—administration & dosage—nurses' instruction.
   2. Drugs—administration & dosage—problems.   3. Problem Solving—
   nurses' instruction.   4. Mathematics—nurses' instruction.   QV 748
   C886c 1997]
   RS57.C73   1997
   615.5'8—dc20
   DNLM/DLC
   for Library of Congress   96-13233
                                                                         CIP

Care has been taken to confirm the accuracy of the information presented and to describe generally accepted practices. However, the authors, editors, and publisher are not responsible for errors or omissions or for any consequences from application of the information in this book and make no warranty, express or implied, with respect to the contents of the publication.

The authors, editors and publisher have exerted every effort to ensure that drug selection and dosage set forth in this text are in accordance with current recommendations and practice at the time of publication. However, in view of ongoing research, changes in government regulations, and the constant flow of information relating to drug therapy and drug reactions, the reader is urged to check the package insert for each drug for any change in indications and dosage and for added warnings and precautions. This is particularly important when the recommended agent is a new or infrequently employed drug.

Some drugs and medical devices presented in this publication have Food and Drug Administration (FDA) clearance for limited use in restricted research settings. It is the responsibility of the health care provider to ascertain the FDA status of each drug or device planned for use in their clinical practice.

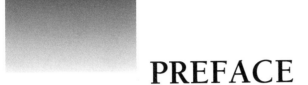

PREFACE

Dosage calculation need not be difficult if you use a problem-solving method that is easy to understand and to implement. Many people experience stumbling blocks calculating mathematical problems because of a lack of mathematical ability or associated mathematical anxiety. Even when this is not the case, many medication errors are made because the medication problems are set up incorrectly. When this happens, there is an increased risk that an incorrect dosage of medication will be administered to the patient, causing extreme consequences to the patient.

As a nontraditional student, I experienced anxiety related to poor mathematical abilities and consequently had difficulty with medication calculations. A friend introduced me to a problem-solving method that was easy for my right brain to visualize. By using this method, I was able to understand all parts of the medication problem and avoid the stumbling blocks that I experienced with other methods of dosage calculation.

Later as a practicing nurse and nursing instructor, I realized that many of my nursing colleagues and my students shared my previous experience associated with low mathematical ability and related "math anxiety." So I began sharing this problem-solving method with other nurses and my students.

This method is **dimensional analysis.** Also called factor-label method and conversion-factor method, dimensional analysis is a systematic, straightforward approach to setting up and solving problems that require conversions. It is a way of *thinking* about problems to be solved and can be used whenever two quantities are directly proportional to each other, but one quantity needs to be converted to the other using a conversion factor before the problem can be solved.

Dimensional analysis provides a framework for understanding the principles of the problem-solving method. It helps the learner to organize and evaluate data, and to avoid errors in setting up the problem. It supports the critical-thinking process. As a problem-solving method, dimensional analysis helps the student with limited mathematical ability and associated anxiety avoid the stumbling blocks that occur when using other math problem-solving approaches such as the ratio and proportion method.

Dimensional analysis empowers the learner to solve a variety of medication problems using just one problem-solving method. This text uses the simple-to-complex approach by providing a review of basic skills required by the learner to use in applying dimensional analysis when solving medication calculation problems. As the learner continues through the text, more complex medication problem-solving examples are presented. Chapter exercises provide an opportunity for the learner to gain ability and build confidence in the material before proceeding to the next chapter. To provide the learner with clinically realistic examples, actual drug labels are liberally used in every chapter as the basis of medication problems.

The Chapter Exercise Answers provides the answer to each problem by showing how the problem was set up and then solved. Finally, the text provides two chapters with a variety of medication problems to assess ability and redirect the learner to the appropriate chapter if difficulty in solving the medication problem is encountered.

Features of the Text:

- Simple-to-complex organization uses sound learning theory
- Step-by-step approach for setting up examples of problem-solving provides clear explanation of how to set up and solve the problem
- In-chapter practice provides ample opportunity for student learning
- Answer key provides easy access and details of problem-solving
- Use of actual drug labels simulates the clinical setting experience
- Special boxes in each chapter, *Thinking Through The Problem,* provide additional guidelines and tips for solving problems

As a method of reducing medication errors and improving medication dosage calculation abilities, dimensional analysis has many possibilities. Regardless of whether it is used in practice or education, dimensional analysis is an approach to use when the goal is improving medication dosage-calculation skills, reducing medication errors, and improving patient safety. Ultimately, this improved methodology might well reduce the medication errors that occur within the discipline of nursing.

Dimensional analysis helps the learner see and understand the significance of the whole process, since it focuses on "how" to learn, rather than "what" to learn. Dimensional analysis supports conceptual mastery and the higher-level thinking skills that have become the core of curriculum change at all levels of nursing education.

During my baccalaureate nursing education, this problem-solving method became my teaching plan. During my master's nursing education, this problem-solving method became my research. Now, I would like to share this problem-solving method with anyone who ever believed that they were mathematically "challenged" or trembled at the thought of solving a medication problem.

Gloria P. Craig

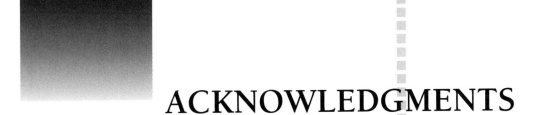

ACKNOWLEDGMENTS

There are many people who have assisted me with my professional growth and development including:

- **Pauline Callahan** who believed that I would be a great nurse and nursing instructor when I could not believe in myself.
- **Jackie Kehm** who introduced me to dimensional analysis and helped me pass the medication module that I was sure would be my stumbling block.
- **Dr. Sandra L. Sellers** for her expertise and guidance throughout the process of writing my thesis and her encouragement to write a textbook.
- **Margaret Cooper** for her friendship and editing support throughout the writing of this textbook.
- My students, colleagues, and reviewers for helping me develop my abilities to explain and teach the problem-solving method of dimensional analysis.
- The numerous pharmaceutical companies listed throughout this book that supplied medication labels and gave permission for the labels to be included in this textbook.
- The Lippincott editorial and production team, for all their hard work: **Margaret Belcher Zuccarini**, Senior Nursing Editor, **Emily Cotlier**, Editorial Assistant, **Barbara Ryalls**, Project Editor, and **Doug Smock**, Assistant Art Director.

To these people and many more, I would like to express my sincere appreciation for their mentoring, guidance, support, and encouragement that have helped to turn a dream into a reality.

CONTENTS

1 Arithmetic Review   1
Arabic Numbers and Roman Numerals   2
Fractions   11
Decimals   17

2 Common Equivalents   27
Systems of Measurement   27

3 Solving Problems With Dimensional Analysis   37
Dimensional Analysis   38

4 One-Factor Medication Problems   51
Interpretation of Medication Orders   52
One-Factor Medication Problems   53
Components of a Drug Label   61
Administering Medication by Different Routes   67

5 Two-Factor Medication Problems   85
Medication Problems Involving Weight   86
Medication Problems Involving Reconstitution   93
Medication Problems Involving Intravenous Pumps   98
Medication Problems Involving Drop Factors   104
Medication Problems Involving Intermittent Infusion   111

6 Three-Factor Medication Problems   117
Medication Problems Involving Dosage, Weight, and Time   118

7   **Practicing Problems With Dimensional Analysis**   137
One-Factor Practice Problems   **137**
Two-Factor Practice Problems   **148**
Three-Factor Practice Problems   **153**

8   **Comprehensive Post-Test**   159

9   **Case Study-Based Clinical Calculations**   165

Appendix   185
Bibliography   199
Glossary   201
Chapter Exercise Answers   203
Index   275

INTRODUCTION

Dimensional analysis is a problem-solving method based on the principles of cognitive theory. Bruner (1960) theorized that learning is dependent on how information is structured, organized, and conceptualized. He proposed a cognitive learning model that emphasized the acquisition, organization (structure), understanding, and transfer of knowledge—focusing on "how" to learn, rather than "what" to learn. Learning involves associations established according to the principles of continuity and repetition.

Dimensional analysis (also called factor-label method, conversion-factor method, units analysis, and quantity calculus) provides a systematic way to set up problems and helps to organize and evaluate data. Hein (1983) emphasized that dimensional analysis gives a clear understanding of the principles of the problem-solving method that correlates with the ability to verbalize what steps are taken leading to critical thinking. He described dimensional analysis as a useful method for solving a variety of chemistry, physics, mathematics, and daily life problems. He identified that dimensional analysis is often the problem-solving method of choice because it provides a straightforward way to set up problems, gives a clear understanding of the principles of the problem, helps the learner to organize and evaluate data, and assists in identifying errors if the setup of the problem is incorrect.

Goodstein (1983) described dimensional analysis as a problem-solving method that is very simple to understand, reduces errors, and requires less conceptual reasoning power to understand than does the ratio–proportion method. She expressed that "even though the ratio–proportion method was at one time the primary problem-solving method, it has been largely replaced by a dimensional analysis approach in most introductory chemistry textbooks . . . this method condenses multi-step problems into one orderly extended solution."

Peters (1986) identified dimensional analysis as a method used for solving not only chemistry problems but also a variety of other mathematical problems that require conversions. He defined dimensional analysis as a method that can be used whenever two quantities are directly proportional to each other and one quantity must be converted to the other using a conversion factor or conversion relationship.

Recent literature that has examined the quality of higher education and professional education in the United States (National Institute of Education, 1984) recommends that educators increase the emphasis of the intellectual skills of problem-solving and critical thinking. Also recommended is an increase on the emphasis of the mastery of concepts rather than specific facts. Other literature on curriculum revolution in nursing (Bevis, 1988; Lindeman, 1989; Tanner, 1988) recommends that learning not be characterized merely as a change in behavior or the acquisition of facts, but in seeing and *understanding* the significance of the whole. Because it focuses on "how" to learn, rather than "what" to learn, dimensional analysis supports conceptual mastery and higher-level thinking skills that have become the core of the curriculum change that is sweeping through all levels of education and, most importantly, nursing education.

Clinical Calculations Using Dimensional Analysis

1 Arithmetic Review

Chapter Objectives

After completing this chapter, the learner will be able to:

1. Express Arabic numbers as Roman numerals.
2. Express Roman numerals as Arabic numbers.
3. Identify the numerator and denominator in a fraction.
4. Multiply and divide fractions.
5. Convert fractions to decimals.
6. Multiply and divide decimals.

Every nurse must know and practice the **five rights of drug administration** including the

1. Right *drug*
2. Right *dose*
3. Right *route*
4. Right *time*
5. Right *patient*

Although the right drug, route, time, and patient may be readily identified, the right *dose* requires arithmetic, conceptual, and cognitive skills that may pose difficulty for some learners.

This chapter will assist learners by reviewing basic arithmetic skills that will prepare them to calculate medication dosage problems using the problem-solving method of **dimensional analysis.**

○ Arabic Numbers and Roman Numerals

Most medication dosages are ordered by the physician in the metric and household systems for weights and measures using the Arabic number system with symbols called **digits** (*ie*, 1, 2, 3, 4, 5). Occasionally, orders are received in the apothecary system of weights and measures using the Roman numeral system with numbers represented by **symbols** (*ie*, I, V, X). The Roman numeral system uses seven basic symbols, and various combinations of these symbols represent all numbers in the Arabic number system.

Box 1-1 includes the seven basic Roman numerals and the corresponding Arabic numbers.

Box 1-1.

Roman Numerals		Arabic Numbers
I	=	1
V	=	5
X	=	10
L	=	50
C	=	100
D	=	500
M	=	1000

The combination of Roman numeral symbols is based on three specific learning principles including:

- Symbols are used to construct a number, but no symbol may be used more than three times. The exception is the symbol for five (V), which is used only once because there is a symbol for 10 (X) and a combination of symbols for 15 (XV).

EXAMPLE: III = (1 + 1 + 1) = 3

EXAMPLE: XXX = (10 + 10 + 10) = 30

- When symbols of lesser value follow symbols of greater value they are *added* to construct a number.

EXAMPLE: VIII = (5 + 3) = 8

EXAMPLE: XVII = (10 + 5 + 1 + 1) = 17

- When symbols of greater value follow symbols of lesser value those of lesser value are *subtracted* from those of higher value to construct a number.

EXAMPLE: IV = (5 − 1) = 4

EXAMPLE: IX = (10 − 1) = 9

Exercise 1

Express the following Arabic numbers as Roman numerals.

1. 1 = _____

2. 2 = _____

3. 3 = _____

4. 4 = _____

5. 5 = _____

6. 6 = _____

7. 7 = _____

8. 8 = _____

9. 9 = _____

10. 10 = _____

11. 11 = _____

12. 12 = _____

13. 13 = _____

14. 14 = _____

15. 15 = _____

16. 16 = _____

17. 17 = _____

18. 18 = _____

19. 19 = _____

20. 20 = _____

Exercise 2

Although medication orders rarely involve Roman numerals higher than 20, for additional practice express the following Arabic numbers as Roman numerals.

1. 43 = _____

2. 24 = _____

3. 55 = _____

4. 32 = _____

5. 102 = _____

6. 150 = _____

7. 75 = _____

8. 92 = _____

9. 64 = _____

10. 69 = _____

Exercise 3

Express the following Roman numerals as Arabic numbers.

1. II = _____

2. IV = _____

3. VI = _____

4. X = _____

5. VIII = _____

6. XIX = _____

7. XX = _____

8. XVIII = _____

9. I = _____

10. XV = _____

11. III = _____

12. V = _____

13. IX = _____

14. VII = _____

15. XI = _____

16. XIV = _____

17. XVI = _____

18. XII   = _____

19. XVII = _____

20. XIII = _____

Exercise 4

To increase your abilities to use either system, convert the following Arabic numbers or Roman numerals.

1. 19 = _____

2. XII = _____

3. 7   = _____

4. IX   = _____

5. IV = _____

6. 11 = _____

7. VIII = _____

8. 16 = _____

9. XX = _____

10. 5 = _____

11. I = _____

12. 18 = _____

13. VI = _____

14. 2 = _____

15. III = _____

16. 10 = _____

17. XIII = _____

18. 14 = _____

19. XV = _____

20. 17 = _____

Exercise 5

For additional practice, convert the following Arabic numbers or Roman numerals.

1. 34 = _____

2. XXII = _____

3. 75 = _____

4. XC = _____

5. 29 = _____

6. XLII = _ _____

7. 56 = _____

8. LXIV = _____

9. 88 = _____

10. CXXI = _____

○ Fractions

Occasionally medication dosages using fractions are ordered by the physician or labeled by the pharmaceutical manufacturer. A **fraction** is a number that represents part of a whole number and contains three parts:

1. **Numerator**—the number on the top portion of the fraction that represents the number of parts of the whole fraction.

2. **Dividing line**—the line separating the top portion of the fraction from the bottom portion of the fraction.

3. **Denominator**—the number on the bottom portion of the fraction that represents the number of parts into which the whole is divided.

EXAMPLE:

$$\frac{3}{4} = \frac{\text{numerator}}{\text{denominator}}$$

When using dimensional analysis to solve medication dosage calculation problems, the learner must be able to identify the numerator and denominator portion of the problem. The learner also must be able to multiply and divide numbers, fractions, and decimals.

The Learning Principle for multiplying fractions:

1. Multiply the numerators.

2. Multiply the denominators.

3. Reduce the product to the lowest possible fraction.

EXAMPLE: $\frac{2}{4} \times \frac{1}{8} = \frac{2}{32} = \frac{1}{16}$

or

$$\frac{2 \text{ (numerator)}}{4 \text{ (denominator)}} \times \frac{1 \text{ (numerator)}}{8 \text{ (denominator)}} = \frac{2 \text{ (numerator)}}{32 \text{ (denominator)}} = \frac{1}{16} \text{ (reduced to lowest possible fraction)}$$

EXAMPLE: $\frac{1}{2} \times \frac{2}{4} = \frac{2}{8} = \frac{1}{4}$

or

$$\frac{1 \text{ (numerator)}}{2 \text{ (denominator)}} \times \frac{2 \text{ (numerator)}}{4 \text{ (denominator)}} = \frac{2 \text{ (numerator)}}{8 \text{ (denominator)}} = \frac{1}{4} \text{ (reduced to lowest possible fraction)}$$

The Learning Principle for dividing fractions:

1. Invert (turn upside down) the divisor portion of the problem (the divisor portion of the problem is the second fraction in the problem).

2. Multiply the two numerators.

3. Multiply the two denominators.

4. Reduce answer to lowest term (fraction or whole number).

EXAMPLE: $\frac{2}{4} \div \frac{1}{8} = \frac{2}{4} \times \frac{8}{1} = \frac{16}{4} = 4$ (answer reduced to lowest term)

or

(inverted fraction)

$$\frac{2 \text{ (numerator)}}{4 \text{ (denominator)}} \div \frac{1 \text{ (numerator)}}{8 \text{ (denominator)}} = \frac{2 \text{ (numerator)} \times 8 \text{ (numerator)} = 16}{4 \text{ (denominator)} \times 1 \text{ (denominator)} = 4} = 4 \text{ (answer reduced to lowest term)}$$

or

$$\frac{2}{4} \div \frac{1}{8} = \frac{2 \times 8 = 16}{4 \times 1 = 4} = 4$$

EXAMPLE: $\frac{1}{2} \div \frac{2}{4} = \frac{1}{2} \times \frac{4}{2} = \frac{4}{4} = 1$

or

$$\underset{\text{2 (denominator)}}{\underset{}{\text{1 (numerator)}}} \div \underset{\text{4 (denominator)}}{\underset{}{\text{2 (numerator)}}} = \frac{\text{1 (numerator)} \times \overset{\text{(inverted fraction)}}{\text{4 (numerator)}} = 4}{\text{2 (denominator)} \times \text{2 (denominator)} = 4} = 1 \text{ (answer reduced to lowest term)}$$

or

$$\frac{1}{2} \div \frac{2}{4} = \frac{1 \times 4 = 4}{2 \times 2 = 4} = 1$$

Exercise 6

To increase your abilities when working with fractions, multiply the following fractions and reduce to the lowest fractional term.

1. $\frac{3}{4} \times \frac{5}{8} =$

2. $\frac{1}{3} \times \frac{4}{9} =$

3. $\frac{2}{3} \times \frac{4}{5} =$

4. $\frac{3}{4} \times \frac{1}{2} =$

5. $\frac{1}{8} \times \frac{4}{5} =$

6. $\frac{2}{3} \times \frac{5}{8} =$

7. $\frac{3}{8} \times \frac{2}{3} =$

8. $\frac{4}{7} \times \frac{2}{4} =$

9. $\frac{4}{5} \times \frac{1}{2} =$

10. $\frac{1}{4} \times \frac{1}{8} =$

Exercise 7

To increase your abilities when working with fractions, divide the following fractions and reduce to the lowest fractional term.

1. $\frac{3}{4} \div \frac{2}{3} =$

2. $\dfrac{1}{9} \div \dfrac{3}{9} =$

3. $\dfrac{2}{3} \div \dfrac{1}{6} =$

4. $\dfrac{1}{5} \div \dfrac{4}{5} =$

5. $\dfrac{3}{6} \div \dfrac{4}{8} =$

6. $\dfrac{5}{8} \div \dfrac{5}{8} =$

7. $\dfrac{1}{8} \div \dfrac{2}{3} =$

8. $\dfrac{1}{5} \div \dfrac{1}{2} =$

Converting Fractions to Decimals

When problem-solving with Dimensional Analysis, medication dosage-calculation problems may frequently contain both fractions and decimals. Some learners may have fraction phobia and prefer to convert fractions to decimals when solving problems. To convert a fraction to a decimal, divide the numerator portion of the fraction by the denominator portion of the fraction.

EXAMPLE: $\dfrac{1}{2}$ *or* $\dfrac{1 \text{ (numerator)}}{2 \text{ (denominator)}} =$ $\dfrac{0.5 = 0.5}{2\overline{)1.0}}$
$\underline{1\,0}$

When dividing fractions, remember to add a decimal point and a zero if the numerator is unable to be divided by the denominator.

EXAMPLE: $\dfrac{3}{4}$ *or* $\dfrac{3 \text{ (numerator)}}{4 \text{ (denominator)}} =$ $\dfrac{0.75 = 0.75}{4\overline{)3.00}}$
$\underline{2\,8}$
20
$\underline{20}$

Exercise 8

To decrease fraction phobia, practice converting the following fractions to decimals.

1. $\dfrac{1}{8} =$

2. $\dfrac{1}{4} =$

3. $\dfrac{2}{5} =$

4. $\dfrac{3}{5} =$

5. $\dfrac{2}{3} =$

6. $\frac{6}{8} =$

7. $\frac{3}{8} =$

8. $\frac{1}{3} =$

9. $\frac{3}{6} =$

10. $\frac{2}{10} =$

○ Decimals

Medication orders are often written using decimals, and pharmaceutical manufacturers may use decimals when labeling medications. Therefore, the learner must understand the learning principles involving decimals and be able to multiply and divide decimals.

- A decimal point is preceded by a zero if not preceded by a number to decrease chance of an error if the decimal point is missed.

EXAMPLE: 0.25

- A decimal point may be preceded by a number and followed by a number.

EXAMPLE: 1.25

- Numbers to the left of the decimal point are *units, tens, hundreds, thousands,* and *ten-thousands.*
- Numbers to the right of the decimal point are *tenths, hundredths, thousandths,* and *ten-thousandths.*

EXAMPLE: 0.2 = 2 tenths

EXAMPLE: 0.05 = 5 hundredths

EXAMPLE: 0.25 = 25 hundredths

EXAMPLE: 1.25 = 1 unit and 25 hundredths

EXAMPLE: 110.25 = one hundred ten units and 25 hundredths

- Decimals may be rounded off. If the number to the right of the decimal is greater than or equal to 5 (≥ 5), round up to the next number.

EXAMPLE: 0.78 = 0.8

- If the number to the right of the decimal is less than 5 (≤ 5), delete the remaining numbers.

EXAMPLE: 0.213 = 0.2

- When multiplying with decimals, the principles of multiplication still apply. The numbers are multiplied in columns, but the number of decimal points are counted and placed in the answer counting places from right to left.

EXAMPLE:
$$
\begin{array}{r}
2.3 \text{ (1 decimal point)} \\
\times 1.5 \text{ (1 decimal point)} \\
\hline
115 \\
230 \\
\hline
3.45
\end{array}
$$

Answer: (2 decimal points added to the answer counting 2 places from the right to left)

- When dividing with decimals, the principles of dividing still apply, except that the dividing number is changed to a whole number by moving the decimal point to the right. The number being divided also changes by accepting the same number of decimal point moves.

EXAMPLE: 1.   0.5)$\overline{0.75}$

  • Move decimal point one place to the right

  2. $\begin{array}{r} 1.5 \\ 5\overline{)7.5} \\ \underline{5} \\ 2\,5 \\ \underline{2\,5} \\ 0 \end{array}$

Answer: 1.5

Exercise 9

Practice rounding off the following decimals to the tenth.

1. 0.75 =

2. 0.88 =

3. 0.44 =

4. 0.23 =

5. 0.67 =

6. 0.27 =

7. 0.98 =

8. 0.92 =

Exercise 10

Practice multiplying the following decimals.

1.
$$\begin{array}{r} 2.5 \\ \times 4.6 \\ \hline \end{array}$$

2.
$$\begin{array}{r} 1.45 \\ \times 0.25 \\ \hline \end{array}$$

3.
$$\begin{array}{r} 3.9 \\ \times 0.8 \\ \hline \end{array}$$

4.
$$\begin{array}{r} 2.56 \\ \times 0.45 \\ \hline \end{array}$$

5.
$$\begin{array}{r} 10.65 \\ \times\ 0.05 \\ \hline \end{array}$$

6.
$$\begin{array}{r} 1.98 \\ \times 3.10 \\ \hline \end{array}$$

Exercise 11

Practice dividing the following decimals and rounding the answer to the tenth.

1. $3.4\overline{)9.6}$

2. $0.25\overline{)12.50}$

3. $0.56\overline{)18.65}$

4. $0.3\overline{)0.192}$

5. $0.4\overline{)12.43}$

6. $0.5\overline{)12.50}$

7. $0.125\overline{)0.25}$

8. $0.08\overline{)0.085}$

This chapter has reviewed basic arithmetic that will assist the learner to successfully implement dimensional analysis as a problem-solving method for medication dosage calculations. To assess your understanding and retention, complete the following chapter practice problems.

Practice Problems

• • • • • • • • • • • • • •

Change the following Arabic numbers to Roman numerals:

1. 2   =

2. 4   =

3. 5   =

4. 14   =

5. 19   =

Change the following Roman numerals to Arabic numbers:

6. VI   =

7. IX   =

8. XII =

9. XVII =

10. XIX =

Multiply the following fractions and reduce the answer to the lowest fractional term.

11. $\frac{3}{4} \times \frac{2}{5} =$

12. $\frac{2}{3} \times \frac{5}{8} =$

13. $\frac{1}{2} \times \frac{2}{3} =$

14. $\frac{7}{8} \times \frac{1}{3} =$

15. $\frac{4}{5} \times \frac{2}{7} =$

Divide the following fractions and reduce the answer to the lowest fractional term.

16. $\frac{1}{2} \div \frac{3}{4} =$

17. $\frac{1}{3} \div \frac{7}{8} =$

18. $\frac{1}{5} \div \frac{1}{2} =$

19. $\frac{4}{8} \div \frac{2}{3} =$

20. $\frac{1}{3} \div \frac{2}{3} =$

Convert the following fractions to decimals and round to the tenth.

21. $\frac{1}{2} =$

22. $\frac{1}{3} =$

23. $\frac{3}{4}$ =

24. $\frac{2}{3}$ =

25. $\frac{1}{8}$ =

Multiply the following decimals:

26. $\begin{array}{r} 6.45 \\ \times 1.36 \\ \hline \end{array}$

27. $\begin{array}{r} 3.14 \\ \times 2.20 \\ \hline \end{array}$

28. $\begin{array}{r} 16.286 \\ \times\ 0.125 \\ \hline \end{array}$

29. $\begin{array}{r} 1.2 \\ \times \underline{0.5} \end{array}$

30. $\begin{array}{r} 7.68 \\ \times \underline{0.05} \end{array}$

Divide the following decimals:

31. $0.5\overline{)1.25}$

32. $0.20\overline{)40.80}$

33. $0.125\overline{)0.25}$

34. $0.75\overline{)0.125}$

35. $0.5\overline{)7.30}$

2

Common Equivalents

Chapter Objectives

After completing this chapter, the learner will be able to:

1. Identify measurements included in the metric, apothecary, and household systems.
2. Understand abbreviations used in the metric, apothecary, and household systems.

Medication calculation need not be difficult if the learner has a problem-solving method that is easy to understand and implement. In addition, the learner needs to understand common equivalents and units of measurement, to visualize all parts of a medication dosage calculation problem. *Dimensional analysis,* by the use of critical thinking, allows conceptualization of a medication dosage calculation problem and visualization of all parts of a problem.

This chapter will help the learner to completely understand the measurement systems used for medication dosage administration. This knowledge is necessary for one to accurately implement the problem-solving method of dimensional analysis.

◯ Systems of Measurement

There are three systems of measurement used for medication dosage administration: the metric system, the apothecary system, and the household system. To be able to accurately administer medication, it is necessary to understand all three of these systems.

> **Box 2-1.** Metric System's Units of Weight and Equivalents
>
> 1 kilogram (kg)
> 1 gram (g)
> 1 milligram (mg)
> 1 microgram (mcg)
> 1 kg = 1000 g
> 1 g = 1000 mg
> 1 mg = 1000 mcg

The **metric system** is a decimal system of weights and measures based on units of ten in which gram, meter, and liter are the basic units of measurement. However, gram and liter are the only measurements from the metric system that are used in medication administration. The gram (abbreviated g or gm) is a unit of weight and the liter (abbreviated L) is a unit of volume. The meter is a unit of distance.

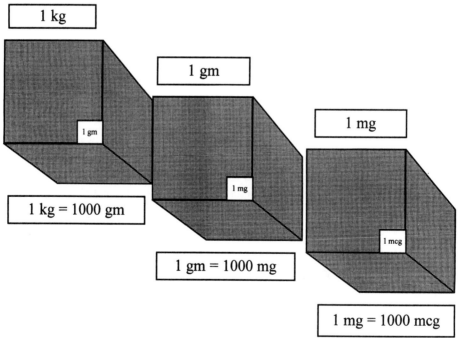

Figure 2-1. Metric system unit of weight and equivalent.

> **Box 2-2.** Metric System's Units of Volume and Equivalents
>
> 1 liter (L)
> 1 milliliter (mL)
> 1 cubic centimeter (cc)
> 1 L = 1000 mL
> 1 mL = 1 cc

The most frequently used metric units of *weight* and their equivalents are summarized in Box 2-1.

Another way to understand the metric units of weight and their equivalents is to visualize the relationship between the measurements and equivalents displayed in Figure 2-1.

The most frequently used metric units for *volume* and their equivalents are summarized in Box 2-2.

Another way to understand the metric units of volume and their equivalents is to visualize the relationship between the measurements and equivalents displayed in Figure 2-2.

Figure 2-2. Metric system unit of volume and equivalent.

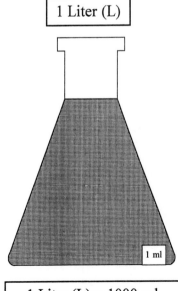

1 Liter (L)

1 Liter (L) = 1000 ml

The **apothecary system** is a system of measuring and weighing drugs and solutions in which fractions are used to identify parts of the unit of measure. The basic units of measurement in the apothecary system include weights and liquid volume. Although this may be replaced by the metric system, it is still necessary to understand it because some physicians continue to order medications using this system, and they also may include Roman numerals in the medication order.

The most frequently used measurements and equivalents within the apothecary units of *weight* are summarized in Box 2-3, and the most frequently used measurements and equivalents within the apothecary system's units of *volume* are summarized in Box 2-4.

The use of household measurements is considered inaccurate because of the varying sizes of cups, glasses, and eating utensils, and this system generally has been replaced with the metric system. However, as patient care moves away from hospitals, which use the metric system, and into the community, it is once again necessary for the nurse to have an understanding of the household measurement system to be able to use and teach it to clients and families.

The most frequently used measurements and equivalents within the household measurement system are summarized in Box 2-5.

Sometimes it is necessary to convert from one system to another to be able to accurately administer medication. Box 2-6 summarizes the most frequently used measurements and lists the approximate equivalents in the metric, apothecary, and household systems.

This chapter has reviewed the metric, apothecary, and household systems of measurement to assist the learner in accurately implementing dimensional analysis as a problem-solving method for medication dosage calculation. To assess your understanding and retention of the systems of measurement, complete the following practice problems.

Box 2-3. Apothecary System's Units of Weight and Equivalents

1 pound (lb)
1 ounce (oz)
1 dram (dr)
1 grain (gr)
1 lb = 16 oz
1 oz = 8 dr
1 dr = 60 gr

Box 2-4. Apothecary System's Units of Volume and Equivalents

1 gallon (gal)
1 quart (qt)
1 pint (pt)
1 fluid ounce (foz) ℥
1 fluid dram (fdr) ℨ
1 minim (M)
1 gal = 4 qt
1 qt = 2 pt
1 pt = 16 foz
1 foz = 8 fdr
1 fdr = 60 M
1 foz = 1 oz
1 fdr = 1 dr

Box 2-5. Household Measurement System and Equivalents

1 glass
1 cup
1 tablespoon (tbsp or T)
1 teaspoon (tsp or t)
1 drop (gtt)
1 glass = 8 ounces (oz)
1 cup = 8 ounces (oz)
2 Tbsp = 1 oz
3 tsp = 1 tbsp
1 tsp = 60 gtt

Box 2-6. Approximate Equivalents

Metric	Apothecary	Household
1 kg = 1000 g	= 2.2 lb	
	1 lb = 16 oz	
1 g = 1000 mg	= 15 gr	
60 mg	= 1 gr	
1 mg = 1000 mcg		
4000 mL	= 1 gal = 4 qt	
1 L = 1000 mL	= 1 qt = 2 pt	
500 mL	= 1 pt = 16 foz	
240 cc	= 8 oz	= 1 glass
180 cc	= 8 oz	= 1 cup
30 cc	= 1 oz = 8 dr	= 2 tbsp
15 cc	= $\frac{1}{2}$ oz = 4 dr	= 1 tbsp = 3 tsp
5 cc	= 1 dr = 60 M	= 1 tsp = 60 gtt
1 mL = 1 cc	= 15 M	= 15 gtts
	1 M	= 1 gtt

Practice Problems

Write the correct abbreviation symbols for the following measurements from the metric system:

1. kilogram   =

2. gram   =

3. milligram   =

4. microgram   =

5. liter   =

6. milliliter   =

7. cubic centimeter =

Write the correct abbreviation symbols for the following measurements from the apothecary system:

1. pound   =

2. ounce   =

3. dram   =

4. grain   =

5. gallon   =

6. quart   =

7. pint   =

8. fluid ounce =

9. fluid dram =

10. minim   =

Write the correct abbreviation symbols for the following measurements from the household system:

1. tablespoon =

2. teaspoon   =

3. drop   =

Identify the correct numerical values for the following measurements:

1.   1 kg = _____ lb

2.   1 kg = _____ g

3.   1 g   = _____ mg

4.   1 mg = _____ mcg

5.   1 g   = _____ gr

6.   1 gr = _____ mg

7. 1000 mg = ＿＿ g

8. 1000 mL = ＿＿ L = ＿＿ qt

9. 500 mL = ＿＿ pt

10. 240 mL = ＿＿ oz

11. 30 mL = ＿＿ oz = ＿＿ tbsp

12. 15 mL = ＿＿ oz = ＿＿ tsp

13. 5 mL = ＿＿ tsp

14. 1 mL = ＿＿ M = ＿＿ gtt

15. 1 mL = ＿＿ cc

3

Solving Problems With Dimensional Analysis

Chapter Objectives

After completing this chapter, the learner will be able to:

1. Define dimensional analysis.
2. Explain step-by-step the problem-solving method of dimensional analysis.
3. Solve problems involving common equivalents using dimensional analysis as a problem-solving method.

Dimensional analysis provides a systematic, straightforward way to set up problems and helps one to organize and evaluate data. Chemistry educators have adopted dimensional analysis as a method that is not only easier to learn, but also reduces errors when some types of mathematical conversion are required. This system, through critical thinking, allows conceptualization of a problem, and use of its concepts supports visualization of all parts of a problem.

This chapter introduces the learner to dimensional analysis with a step-by-step explanation of this problem-solving method. The chapter will also provide the learner the opportunity to practice solving problems that involve common equivalents by using this method and thereby enhance learning.

◯ Dimensional Analysis

Dimensional analysis is a problem-solving method that can be used whenever two quantities are directly proportional to each other and one quantity must be converted to the other by using a common equivalent, conversion factor, or conversion relation. Once the beginning point in the problem is identified, then a series of conversions necessary to achieve the answer is established that leads to the problem's solution.

It is important to understand the following four terms that provide the basis for dimensional analysis. With these four terms, all medication dosage calculation problems can be solved by dimensional analysis. These terms include the following:

- **Given quantity:** the beginning point of the problem.

- **Wanted quantity:** the answer to the problem.

- **Unit path:** the series of conversions necessary to achieve the answer to the problem.

- **Conversion factors:** equivalents necessary to convert between systems of measurement and to allow unwanted units to be canceled from the problem.

Below is an example of the problem-solving method, showing the placement of basic terms used in dimensional analysis.

	Unit Path			
Given Quantity	Conversion Factor For Given Quantity	Conversion Factor For Wanted Quantity	Conversion Computation	Wanted Quantity
1 liter (L)	1000 mL / 1 liter (L)	1 oz / 30 mL	$\dfrac{1 \times 1000 \times 1\ oz}{1 \times 30}$ $\dfrac{1000}{30}$	= 33.3 ounces

Once the given quantity is identified, the unit path leading to the wanted quantity is established. The problem-solving method of dimensional analysis can be explained using the following five steps.

1. Identify the *given quantity* in the problem.

2. Identify the *wanted quantity* in the problem.

3. Establish the *unit path* from the given quantity to the wanted quantity using equivalents as *conversion factors*.

4. Set up the problem to permit cancellation of unwanted units.

5. Multiply the numerators, multiply the denominators, and divide the product of the numerators by the product of the denominators to provide the numerical value of the wanted quantity.

The following example uses the five steps to solve a problem using dimensional analysis.

EXAMPLE #1:   1 liter (L) equals how many ounces (oz):
Or: How many ounces are in 1 L?

Step #1:   Identify the *given quantity* in the problem.

Need to know: What is the given quantity?

Answer: The given quantity is *1 L.*

Unit Path

Given Quantity	Conversion Factor For Given Quantity	Conversion Factor For Wanted Quantity	Conversion Computation	Wanted Quantity
1 liter (L)				=

Step #2:   Identify the *wanted quantity* in the problem.

Need to know: What is the wanted quantity?

Answer: The wanted quantity is the number of *ounces* (oz) in 1 L.

Unit Path

Given Quantity	Conversion Factor For Given Quantity	Conversion Factor For Wanted Quantity	Conversion Computation	Wanted Quantity
1 liter (L)				= oz

• • • • • THINKING THROUGH THE PROBLEM

Dimensional analysis is a problem-solving method that uses the same terms as fractions, specifically numerators and denominators.

the *numerator* = the top portion of the problem

the *denominator* = the bottom portion of the problem.

Some problems will have a given quantity and a wanted quantity that contain only numerators. Other problems will have a given quantity and a wanted quantity that contain both a numerator and a denominator. This chapter contains only problems with numerators as the given quantity and the wanted quantity.

Step #3: Establish the *unit path* from the given quantity to the wanted quantity by selecting the equivalents that will be used as conversion factors.

Need to know: What conversion factors are needed in the unit path that will convert the given quantity to the wanted quantity?

Answer: given quantity of 1 L = 1000 mL
wanted quantity of 1 oz = 30 mL

Unit Path

Given Quantity	Conversion Factor For Given Quantity	Conversion Factor For Wanted Quantity	Conversion Computation		Wanted Quantity
1 liter (L)	1000 mL	1 oz			
	1 liter (L)	30 mL		=	oz

Step #4: Write the unit path for the problem so that each unit cancels out the preceding unit until all unwanted units are canceled from the problem except the wanted quantity.

Need to know: What is the wanted quantity that remains in the unit path after canceling all unwanted units?

Answer:

Unit Path

Given Quantity	Conversion Factor For Given Quantity	Conversion Factor For Wanted Quantity	Conversion Computation		Wanted Quantity
1 liter (L)	1000 ~~mL~~	1 (oz)			
	1 ~~liter (L)~~	30 ~~mL~~		=	oz

• • • • • • **THINKING THROUGH THE PROBLEM**

> Each conversion factor is a ratio of units that equals 1. The conversion factors are set up to cancel out the preceding unit. The wanted quantity must be within the numerator portion of the problem to identify that the problem is set up correctly. Carefully choose each conversion factor and ensure that it is correctly placed in the numerator or denominator portion of the problem to allow the unwanted units to be canceled from the problem. If you are unable to cancel unwanted units because both units are numerators or denominators, then the problem is not set up correctly. The units need to be opposite each other to be canceled from the problem.

Step #5: After the unwanted units are canceled from the problem, only the numerical values remain. Multiply the numerators, multiply the denominators, and divide the product of the numerators by the product of the denominators to provide the numerical value for the wanted quantity.

Need to know:

• What is the product of the numerators?

• What is the product of the denominators?

• After multiplying the numerators and the denominators, and dividing the product of the numerators by the product of the denominators, what is the numerical value for the wanted quantity?

Answer: The wanted quantity is 33.3 oz and the answer to the problem.

Unit Path

Given Quantity	Conversion Factor For Given Quantity	Conversion Factor For Wanted Quantity	Conversion Computation	Wanted Quantity
1 L̶	1000 m̶L̶	1 (oz)	1000 × 1 oz	$\dfrac{1000}{30} = 33.3$ oz
	1 l̶i̶t̶e̶r̶ (L̶)	30 m̶L̶	30	

• • • • • THINKING THROUGH THE PROBLEM

Ounces is the wanted quantity in the problem and is the remaining unit left in the problem after the unwanted units are canceled from the problem. Ounces is correctly placed in the numerator portion of the problem to correspond with the wanted quantity in the numerator portion of the problem.

Another example of the problem-solving method of dimensional analysis is summarized as follows:

EXAMPLE #2:   One gallon (gal) equals how many milliliters?
Or: How many milliliters are in 1 gal?

Step #1:   Identify the given quantity in the problem.

Need to know: What is the given quantity?

Answer: The given quantity is 1 gal.

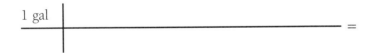

Step #2:   Identify the wanted quantity in the problem.

Need to know: What is the wanted quantity?

Answer: The wanted quantity is the number of *milliliters* (ml) in 1 gal.

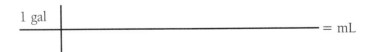

Step #3:   Establish the unit path from the given quantity to the wanted quantity by selecting the equivalents that will be used as conversion factors.

Need to know: What conversion factors are needed in the unit path that will convert the given quantity to the wanted quantity?

Answer:

Given quantity of 1 gal = 4 quarts (qt)

$$1 \text{ qt} = 1 \text{ L}$$

$$1 \text{ L} = 1000 \text{ mL the wanted quantity unit}$$

Step #4: Write the unit path for the problem so that each unit cancels out the preceding unit until all unwanted units are canceled from the problem except the wanted quantity.

Need to know: What is the wanted quantity that remains in the unit path after canceling all unwanted units?

Answer:

$$\frac{1 \text{ gal} \mid 4 \text{ qt} \mid 1 \text{ L} \mid 1000 \text{ (mL)}}{\mid 1 \text{ gal} \mid 1 \text{ qt} \mid 1 \text{ L}} = \quad \text{mL}$$

Step #5: After the unwanted units are canceled from the problem, only the numerical values remain. Multiply the numerators, multiply the denominators, and divide the product of the numerators by the product of the denominators to provide the numerical value for the wanted quantity.

Need to know:

• What is the product of the numerators?

• What is the product of the denominators?

• After multiplying the numerators and the denominators, and dividing the product of the numerators by the product of the denominators, what is the numerical value for the wanted quantity?

Answer:

$$\frac{1 \text{ gal} \mid 4 \text{ qt} \mid 1 \text{ L} \mid 1000 \text{ (mL)} \mid 4 \times 1000}{\mid 1 \text{ gal} \mid 1 \text{ qt} \mid 1 \text{ L} \mid 1} = 4000 \text{ mL}$$

• • • • • THINKING THROUGH THE PROBLEM

One (1) times (×) any number equals that number, therefore 1s may be automatically canceled from the problem. Other factors that can be canceled from the problem include like numerical values in the numerator and denominator portion of the problem and the same number of zeroes in the numerator and denominator portion of the problem.

Exercise 1

Use dimensional analysis to change the following units of measurement.

1. Problem: 4 mg = How many g?

   Given quantity   =

   Wanted quantity   =

   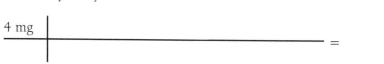

   = g

2. Problem: 5000 g = How many kg?

   Given quantity   =

   Wanted quantity   =

   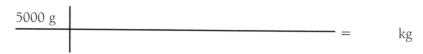

   = kg

3. Problem: 0.3 L = How many cc?

   Given quantity   =

   Wanted quantity   =

   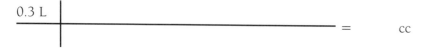

   = cc

4. Problem: 10 cc = How many mL?

Given quantity   =

Wanted quantity   =

$$\frac{10\ cc}{\rule{3cm}{0pt}} = \quad mL$$

5. Problem: 120 lb = How many kg?

Given quantity   =

Wanted quantity   =

$$\frac{120\ lb}{\rule{3cm}{0pt}} = \quad kg$$

6. Problem: 5 gr = How many mg?

Given quantity   =

Wanted quantity   =

$$\frac{5\ gr}{\rule{3cm}{0pt}} = \quad mg$$

7. Problem: 2 g = How many gr?

Given quantity   =

Wanted quantity =

$$\frac{2\ g}{\rule{3cm}{0pt}} = \quad gr$$

8. Problem: 5 fdr = How many mL?

Given quantity   =

Wanted quantity   =

$$\frac{5 \text{ fdr}}{} = \quad \text{mL}$$

9. Problem: 8 fdr = How many foz?

Given quantity   =

Wanted quantity   =

$$\frac{8 \text{ fdr}}{} = \quad \text{foz}$$

10. Problem: 10 M = How many fdr?

Given quantity   =

Wanted quantity   =

$$\frac{10 \text{ M}}{} = \quad \text{fdr}$$

11. Problem: 35 kg = How many lb?

Given quantity   =

Wanted quantity   =

$$\frac{35 \text{ kg}}{} = \quad \text{lb}$$

12. Problem: 10 mL = How many tsp?

Given quantity   =

Wanted quantity   =

   = ___ tsp

13. Problem: 30 mL = How many tbsp?

Given quantity   =

Wanted quantity   =

$$\frac{30 \text{ mL}}{} = \text{___ tbsp}$$

14. Problem: 0.25 g = How many mg?

Given quantity   =

Wanted quantity   =

$$\frac{0.25 \text{ g}}{} = \text{___ mg}$$

15. Problem: 350 mcg = How many mg?

Given quantity   =

Wanted quantity   =

$$\frac{350 \text{ mcg}}{} = \text{___ mg}$$

16. Problem: 0.75 L = How many mL?

    Given quantity   =

    Wanted quantity   =

    $$\frac{0.75\ L}{\rule{4cm}{0pt}} = \quad mL$$

17. Problem: 3 hr = How many minutes?

    Given quantity   =

    Wanted quantity   =

    $$\frac{3\ hr}{\rule{4cm}{0pt}} = \quad min$$

18. Problem: 3.5 mL = How many M?

    Given quantity   =

    Wanted quantity   =

    $$\frac{3.5\ mL}{\rule{4cm}{0pt}} = \quad M$$

19. Problem: 500 mcg = How many mg?

    Given quantity   =

    Wanted quantity   =

    $$\frac{500\ mcg}{\rule{4cm}{0pt}} = \quad mg$$

20. Problem: 225 M = How many tsp?

Given quantity   =

Wanted quantity   =

$$\frac{225 \text{ M} \quad |}{\rule{8cm}{0pt}} = \quad \text{tsp}$$

This chapter has introduced the learner to the problem-solving method of dimensional analysis with a step-by-step explanation and an opportunity to practice solving problems involving common equivalents. To demonstrate your understanding of dimensional analysis and conversions between systems of measurement, complete the following practice problems.

Practice Problems

1. Problem: $\frac{3}{4}$ mL   = How many M?

2. Problem: gtt XV = How many M?

3. Problem: $\frac{5}{6}$ gr   = How many mg?

4. Problem: How many mL in 3 oz?

5. Problem: 0.5 mg = How many mcg?

6. Problem: 35 gtt = How many mL?

7. Problem: How many cc in 3 qt?

8. Problem: 4 gal = How many qt?

9. Problem: 1.5 cup = How many cc?

10. Problem: 24 oz = How many glasses?

4

One-Factor Medication Problems

Chapter Objectives

After completing this chapter the learner will be able to:

1. Interpret medication orders correctly, based on the five rights of medication administration.
2. Identify the important components from a drug label that are needed for accurate medication administration.
3. Understand the different routes of medication administration, including tablets and capsules, liquids given by medicine cup or syringe, and parenteral injections using different types of syringes.
4. Accurately calculate medication problems from the one-factor–given quantity to the one-factor–wanted quantity by using the sequential method or the random method of dimensional analysis.

For accurate administration of medication, the "five rights of medication administration" form the foundation of communication between the physician and the nurse. The physician writes a medication order using the five rights, and the nurse administers the medication to the patient based on the five rights. There may be a slight variation in the way each physician writes a medication order, but information pertaining to the five rights should be included in the medication order to ensure safe administration by the nurse.

To calculate the change from a one-factor–given quantity to a one-factor–wanted quantity by dimensional analysis in medication problems, it is necessary to have a clear understanding of the five rights. This chapter will assist the learner to interpret medication orders correctly and to calculate medication problems accurately using dimensional analysis as a problem-solving method.

○ Interpretation of Medication Orders

Physicians order medications by using the five rights of medication administration, which include the

1. Right **patient** (person receiving the medication)
2. Right **drug** (name of the medication)
3. Right **dosage** (amount of medication to be given)
4. Right **route** (how the medication is to be given)
5. Right **time** (when and how often the medication is to be given)

In the following medication orders, identify the five rights of medication administration.

Medication Order #1

Give gr 10 aspirin to Mrs. C. Clark orally every 4 hours, as needed for fever.

1. Right patient   _____
2. Right drug   _____
3. Right dosage   _____
4. Right route   _____
5. Right time   _____

Medication Order #2

Administer PO to Mr. S. Smith, Advil (ibuprofen) 400 mg every 6 hours for arthritis.

1. Right patient   _____
2. Right drug   _____
3. Right dosage   _____
4. Right route   _____
5. Right time   _____

Medication Order #3

Tylenol (acetaminophen) gr 10 PO every 4 hours for Mr. J. Jones prn for headache.

1. Right patient   _____

2. Right drug   _____

3. Right dosage   _____

4. Right route   _____

5. Right time   _____

Once the ability to interpret the important components of an order for medication has been achieved, accurate calculations for the correct drug dosage by dimensional analysis can be performed.

○ One-Factor Medication Problems

The first step in interpreting any physician's order for medication is to identify the *given quantity,* or the exact dosage, of medication that the physician has ordered. The second step is to identify the *wanted quantity,* or the answer to the medication problem. The third step is to establish the *unit path* from the given quantity to the wanted quantity using equivalents as *conversion factors* to complete the problem. Identification of the available dosage of medication (dose on hand) is considered part of the unit path. The fourth step is to set up the problem to cancel out unwanted units, and the fifth step is to multiply numerators, multiply denominators, and divide the product of the numerators by the product of the denominators to provide the *numerical value* of the wanted quantity or the answer to the problem.

By using these five steps, all medication problems can be solved by implementing either the *sequential method* or the *random method* of *dimensional analysis.*

Below is an example of a one-factor problem showing the placement of basic terms used in dimensional analysis.

Unit Path

Given Quantity	Conversion Factor For Given Quantity	Conversion Computation		Wanted Quantity
10 ~~gr~~	tablets	10		
	5 gr	5	=	2 tablets
	Conversion Factor For Wanted Quantity			

Problem Example #1

The physician orders gr 10 aspirin orally every 4 hours, as needed for fever. The unit dose of medication on hand is gr 5 per tablet (5 gr/tab). How many tablets will you administer?

Given quantity   = 10 gr

Wanted quantity = tablets

Dose on hand   = 5 gr/tab

Step #1.   Identify the given quantity (the physician's order).

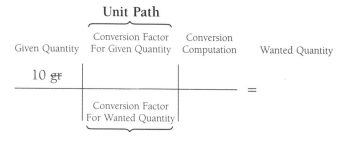

Step #2.   Identify the wanted quantity (the answer to the problem).

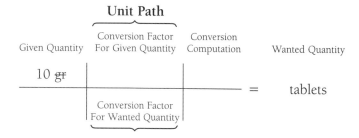

• • • • • THINKING THROUGH THE PROBLEM

10 gr is a numerator without a denominator and *tablets* is a numerator without a denominator. This is called a **one-factor** medication problem because the given quantity and the wanted quantity contain only numerators.

Step #3. Establish the unit path from the given quantity to the wanted quantity using equivalents as conversion factors.

Unit Path

Given Quantity	Conversion Factor For Given Quantity	Conversion Computation	Wanted Quantity
10 g̶r̶	tablets		tablets
	5 gr		
	Conversion Factor For Wanted Quantity		

$$\frac{10\ \text{gr} \quad \text{tablets}}{5\ \text{gr}} = \text{tablets}$$

● ● ● ● ● **THINKING THROUGH THE PROBLEM**

The dose on hand (5 gr/tablets) is an equivalent that is used as a conversion factor and is factored into the unit path.

Step #4. Set up the problem to allow cancellation of unwanted units.

Unit Path

Given Quantity	Conversion Factor For Given Quantity	Conversion Computation	Wanted Quantity
10 g̶r̶	(tablets)		tablets
	5 g̶r̶		
	Conversion Factor For Wanted Quantity		

$$\frac{10\ \text{gr} \quad (\text{tablets})}{5\ \text{gr}} = \text{tablets}$$

● ● ● ● ● **THINKING THROUGH THE PROBLEM**

The unwanted units (gr) can be canceled from the problem leaving the wanted quantity (tablets) in the numerator portion of the unit path, which has been identified as the correct placement of the wanted quantity. The *sequential method* of dimensional analysis has been used to factor in (incorporate into the problem) the dose on hand, which allows the previous unit (given quantity) to be canceled from the unit path. When using the sequential method of dimensional analysis, the conversion factor that is factored into the unit path always cancels out the preceding unit.

Step #5.   Multiply the numerators, multiply the denominators, and divide the product of the numerators by the product of the denominators to provide the numerical value for the wanted quantity.

Unit Path

Given Quantity	Conversion Factor For Given Quantity	Conversion Computation	Wanted Quantity
10 gr	(tablets)	10	
	5 gr	5	= 2 tablets
	Conversion Factor For Wanted Quantity		

2 tablets is the wanted quantity and the answer to the problem.

Problem Example #2

Administer PO Advil (ibuprofen), 400 mg every 6 hours, for arthritis. The dosage on hand is 200 mg/tablet. How many tablets will you give?

Given quantity   = 400 mg

Wanted quantity = tablets

Dose on hand   = 200 mg/tablet

Step #1.   Identify the given quantity.

$$\frac{400 \text{ mg}}{} \qquad\qquad\qquad =$$

Step #2.   Identify the wanted quantity.

$$\frac{400 \text{ mg}}{} \qquad\qquad\qquad = \text{tablets}$$

Step #3.   Establish the unit path from the given quantity to the wanted quantity using equivalents as conversion factors.

$$\frac{400 \text{ mg}}{} \quad \frac{\text{tablet}}{200 \text{ mg}} \qquad\qquad = \text{tablets}$$

Step #4.   Set up the problem to allow cancellation of unwanted units.

$$\frac{400 \; \cancel{mg} \;|\; tablet}{|\; 200 \; \cancel{mg}} = tablets$$

Step #5.   Multiply the numerators, multiply the denominators, and divide the product of the numerators by the product of the denominators to provide the numerical value of the wanted quantity.

$$\frac{\cancel{400} \; \cancel{mg} \;|\; \boxed{tablet} \;|\; 4}{|\; \cancel{200} \; \cancel{mg} \;|\; 2} = 2 \; tablets$$

• • • • • **THINKING THROUGH THE PROBLEM**

> The sequential method of dimensional analysis has been used to set up the problem. The unwanted units (mg) have been canceled from the unit path by correctly factoring in the dose on hand (200 mg/tablet). The same number of zeroes has also been canceled from the numerator and denominator portions of the unit path.

2 tablets is the wanted quantity and the answer to the problem.

Problem Example #3

Tylenol (acetaminophen) gr 10 PO every 4 hours for headache. The unit dose of medication on hand is 325 mg per caplet. How many caplets will you give?

Given quantity   = 10 gr

Wanted quantity = caplets

Dose on hand   = 325 mg/caplet

Step #1.   Identify the given quantity.

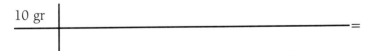

Step #2.   Identify the wanted quantity.

$$\frac{10 \text{ gr}}{\rule{2cm}{0pt}} = \text{caplets}$$

Step #3. Establish the unit path from the given quantity to the wanted quantity using equivalents as conversion factors.

$$\frac{10 \text{ gr} \mid 60 \text{ mg} \mid \text{caplet}}{\mid 1 \text{ gr} \mid 325 \text{ mg}} = \text{caplets}$$

Step #4. Set up the problem to allow cancellation of unwanted units.

$$\frac{10 \text{ g\!r} \mid 60 \text{ m\!g} \mid \boxed{\text{caplet}}}{\mid 1 \text{ g\!r} \mid 325 \text{ m\!g}} = \text{caplets}$$

• • • • • THINKING THROUGH THE PROBLEM

The sequential method of dimensional analysis has been used to set up the problem. The unwanted unit (gr) has been canceled from the unit path by correctly factoring in a conversion factor (1 gr = 60 mg). The dose on hand (325 mg/caplet) is factored into the unit path, which allows the unwanted unit (mg) to be canceled from the problem. The remaining unit (caplet) is in the numerator portion of the problem and correctly correlates with the wanted quantity in the numerator portion of the problem.

Step #5. Multiply the numerators, multiply the denominators, and divide the product of the numerators by the product of the denominators to provide the numerical value of the wanted quantity.

$$\frac{10 \text{ g\!r} \mid 60 \text{ m\!g} \mid \boxed{\text{caplet}} \mid 10 \times 60}{\mid 1 \text{ g\!r} \mid 325 \text{ m\!g} \mid 1 \times 325} \; \frac{600}{325} = 1.8 \text{ caplets}$$

1.8 caplets is the wanted quantity and the answer to the problem, but by using the "rounding off and up" rule, 2 caplets would be given.

• • • • • THINKING THROUGH THE PROBLEM

Dimensional analysis is a problem-solving method that uses critical think-ing and is not a specific formula. Therefore, the important concept to re-member is that *all* unwanted units must be canceled from the unit path. The *random method* of dimensional analysis also can be used when solving medication problems. When using the random method of dimen-sional analysis, the focus is on the correct placement of the conversion factor to correlate with the wanted quantity in the numerator portion of the unit path, without considering the preceding units.

The random method of dimensional analysis will be used to calculate the answer for the previous Problem Example 3.

Step #1. Identify the given quantity.

$$\frac{10 \text{ gr}}{\rule{5cm}{0pt}} =$$

Step #2. Identify the wanted quantity.

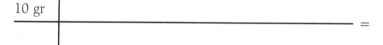

Step #3. Establish the unit path from the given quantity to the wanted quantity using equiv-alents as conversion factors.

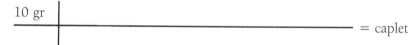

• • • • • THINKING THROUGH THE PROBLEM

When using the random method of dimensional analysis, the focus is on the correct placement of the conversion factor in the unit path to corre-spond with the wanted quantity. The problem is set up correctly as long as the dose on hand (caplet) is in the numerator portion of the unit path to correlate with the wanted quantity (caplet) that also is in the numera-tor portion of the unit path.

Step #4. Set up the problem to allow cancellation of unwanted units.

$$\frac{10 \text{ gr} \mid \cancel{\text{(caplet)}} \mid 60 \text{ mg}}{\mid 325 \text{ mg} \mid 1 \text{ gr}} = \text{caplet}$$

• • • • • THINKING THROUGH THE PROBLEM

A conversion factor (1 gr = 60 mg) is factored into the problem to cancel out the unwanted units (gr and mg) in the unit path. The remaining
unit in the unit path (caplet) correctly correlates with the wanted quantity
in the numerator portion of the problem.

Step #5. Multiply the numerators, multiply the denominators, and divide the product of
the numerators by the product of the denominators to provide the numerical value
of the wanted quantity.

$$\frac{10 \text{ gr} \mid \text{(caplet)} \mid 60 \text{ mg} \mid 10 \times 60 \mid 600}{\mid 325 \text{ mg} \mid 1 \text{ gr} \mid 325 \times 1 \mid 325} = 1.8 \text{ caplets}$$

1.8 caplets is the wanted quantity, and the answer to the problem, but by using the rounding off and up rule, 2 caplets would be given.

Practice Problems
• • • • • • • • • • • • • •

1. The physician orders Achromycin (tetracycline) 0.25 g PO every 12 hours for acne. The
dosage of medication on hand is 250 mg per capsule. How many capsules will you
give?

2. Administer phenobarbital gr $\frac{1}{2}$ PO tid for sedation. The dosage on hand is 15 mg/tablet.
How many tablets will you give?

3. Give 0.5 g Diuril PO bid for hypertension. Unit dose is 500 mg per tablet. How many
tablets will you give?

4. Order: Restoril 0.03 g PO hs for sedation.
Supply: Restoril 30 mg capsules.

5. Order: Thorazine gr $\frac{1}{2}$ PO tid for singultus.
Supply: Thorazine 30 mg spansules.

⊖ **Components of a Drug Label**

All medications are labeled with a drug label that includes specific information, whether it is stock or unit-dose medication, to assist in the accurate administration of the medication. Information on the drug label includes

- Name of the drug, including the trade name (name given by the pharmaceutical company identified with a trademark symbol) and the generic name (chemical name given to the drug)

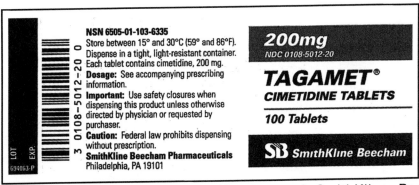

Figure 4-1. Tagamet®/cimetidine. (Courtesy of SmithKline Beecham Pharmaceuticals)

- The dosage of medication (the amount of medication in each tablet, capsule, or liquid)
- The form of medication (tablet, capsule, or liquid)
- The expiration date (how long the medication will remain stable and safe to administer)
- The lot number (the manufacturer's batch series that the medication came from)
- The manufacturer (the pharmaceutical company that produced the medication)

Once the ability to identify the important components of a drug label has been achieved, one's ability to use critical thinking and to solve problems by dimensional analysis can be performed to accurately calculate medication problems.

Drug Label Problem #1

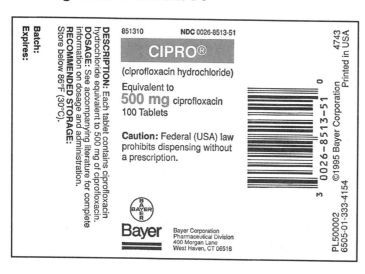

Figure 4-2. Cipro®/ciprofloxacin hydrochloride. (Courtesy of Bayer Corporation Pharmaceutical Division)

The physician orders Cipro, 750 mg PO every 12 hours, for a bacterial infection. How many tablets will you give?

Given quantity = 750 mg

Wanted quantity = tablets

Dose on hand = 500 mg/tablet

Sequential method:

$$\frac{750 \text{ mg} \mid \text{tablet} \mid 75}{\mid 500 \text{ mg} \mid 50} = 1.5 \text{ tablets}$$

1.5 tablets is the wanted quantity and the answer to the problem.

• • • • • THINKING THROUGH THE PROBLEM

The wanted quantity and the answer to the problem is 1.5 tablets. It is possible to administer 1.5 tablets because a scored tablet can be cut in half allowing the exact dosage to be administered.

Drug Label Problem #2

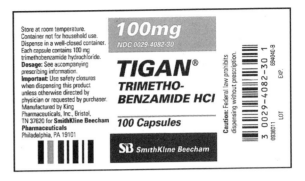

Figure 4-3. Tigan®/trimethobenzamide hydro-chloride. (Courtesy of SmithKline Beecham Pharmaceuticals)

Administer Tigan, 200 mg PO qid, for nausea. How many capsules will you give?

Given quantity   = 200 mg

Wanted quantity = capsules

Dose on hand   = 100 mg/capsules

Sequential method:

$$\frac{200 \text{ mg} \left| \text{capsules} \right| 2}{\left| 100 \text{ mg} \right| 1} = 2 \text{ capsules}$$

The wanted quantity and answer to the problem is 2 capsules.

Drug Label Problem #3

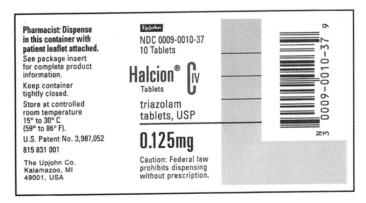

Figure 4-4. Halcion®/triazolam. (Courtesy of the Upjohn Company)

Order: Halcion, 0.25 mg PO hs prn. How many tablets will you give?

Given quantity   = 0.25 mg

Wanted quantity = tablets

Dose on hand   = 0.125 mg/tablet

Sequential method:

$$\frac{0.25 \; \text{mg}}{} \left| \; \text{tablet} \; \right| \frac{0.25}{0.125 \; \text{mg} \; 0.125} = 2 \; \text{tablets}$$

The wanted quantity and the answer to the problem is 2 tablets.

Practice Problems with Drug Labels

1. Order: Compazine, 10 mg PO qid for psychoses.
   How many tablets will you give?

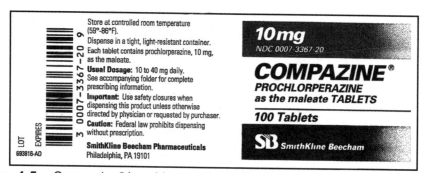

Figure 4-5. Compazine®/prochlorperazine. (Courtesy of SmithKline Beecham Pharmaceuticals)

2. Order: Xanax, 500 mcg PO bid for anxiety.
   How many tablets will you give?

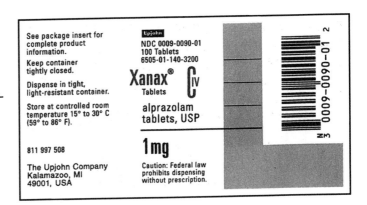

Figure 4-6. Xanax®/alprazolam. (Courtesy of the Upjohn Company)

3. Order: Tolinase, 375 mg PO every AM ac for type II diabetes mellitus.
   How many tablets will you give?

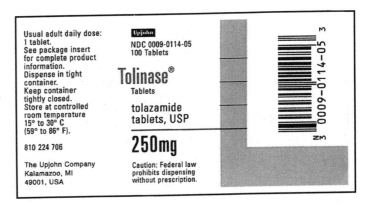

Figure 4-7. Tolinase®/tolazamide. (Courtesy of the Upjohn Company)

4. Order: vitamin B$_{12}$, 2.5 mg daily as a daily vitamin supplement.
How many tablets will you give?

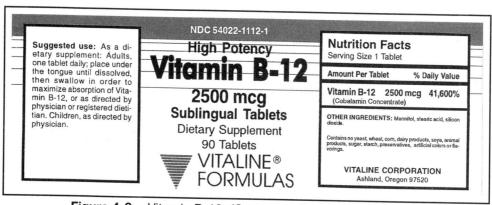

Figure 4-8. Vitamin B-12. (Courtesy of Vitaline Corporation)

5. Order: Tigan, 250 mg PO qid prn for nausea.
How many capsules will you give?

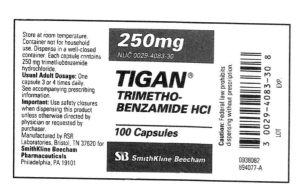

Figure 4-9. Tigan®/trimethobenzamide HCl. (Courtesy of SmithKline Beecham Pharmaceuticals)

○ **Administering Medication by Different Routes**

Medication may be administered by various routes, including oral, parenteral, or intravenous, involving tablets, capsules, or liquid. Oral (PO) medications are administered using tablets, caplets, capsules, or liquid. Tablets and caplets may be scored, which permits a more accurate administration when one-fourth or one-half of a tablet must be given.

Tablets and caplets may also be enteric-coated, which allows the medication to bypass disintegration in the stomach, which will decrease irritation, and then later break down in the small intestine for absorption. Enteric-coated tablets and caplets should never be crushed, because such medications irritate the stomach.

Capsules are usually of the time-released type, and these should never be crushed or opened because the medication would be immediately released into the system, instead of being released slowly over time.

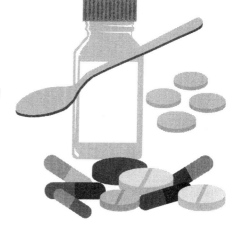

Figure 4-10. Examples of tablets, caplets, capsules, and liquid medicine.

Liquid medication is accurately administered using a medication cup or medication syringe. The medication cup contains the common equivalents for the metric, apothecary, and household systems to permit adaptation of the medication's dosage for administration under various circumstances.

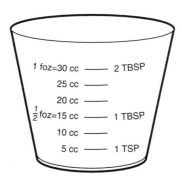

Drug Label Problem #4

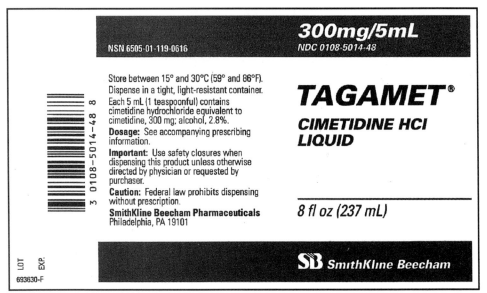

NSN 6505-01-119-0616

300mg/5mL
NDC 0108-5014-48

Store between 15° and 30°C (59° and 86°F).
Dispense in a tight, light-resistant container.
Each 5 mL (1 teaspoonful) contains
cimetidine hydrochloride equivalent to
cimetidine, 300 mg; alcohol, 2.8%.
Dosage: See accompanying prescribing
information.
Important: Use safety closures when
dispensing this product unless otherwise
directed by physician or requested by
purchaser.
Caution: Federal law prohibits dispensing
without prescription.
SmithKline Beecham Pharmaceuticals
Philadelphia, PA 19101

TAGAMET®

**CIMETIDINE HCl
LIQUID**

8 fl oz (237 mL)

3 0108-5014-48 8

SB SmithKline Beecham

LOT   EXP.
693630-F

Figure 4-11. Tagamet®/cimetidine HCl. (Courtesy of SmithKline Beecham Pharmaceuticals)

Order: Tagamet 600 mg PO bid for gastrointestinal (GI) bleeding. How many tsp will you give?

Given quantity   = 600 mg

Wanted quantity = tsp

Dose on hand   = 300 mg/5 mL

Sequential method:

$$\frac{600 \text{ mg}}{} \begin{array}{|c|c|c|c|} 5 \text{ mL} & \text{(tsp)} & 6 \times 5 & 30 \\ \hline 300 \text{ mg} & 5 \text{ mL} & 3 \times 5 & 15 \end{array} = 2 \text{ tsp}$$

The wanted quantity and the answer to the problem is 2 tsp.

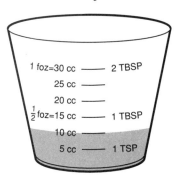

1 foz=30 cc ——— 2 TBSP
25 cc ———
20 cc ———
½ foz=15 cc ——— 1 TBSP
10 cc ———
5 cc ——— 1 TSP

Drug Label Problem #5

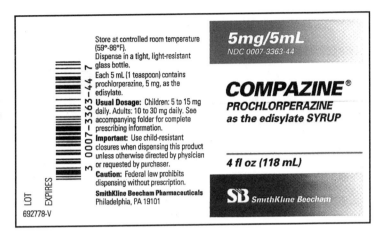

Figure 4-12. Compazine®/prochlorperazine. (Courtesy of SmithKline Beecham Pharmaceuticals)

Order: Compazine 10 mg PO qid for psychomotor agitation. How many mL will you give?

Given quantity   = 10 mg

Wanted quantity = mL

Dose on hand   = 5 mg/5 mL

Sequential Method:

$$\frac{10 \text{ mg} \mid 5 \text{ (mL)} \mid 10}{\mid 5 \text{ mg} \mid} = 10 \text{ mL}$$

The wanted quantity and the answer to the problem is 10 mL.

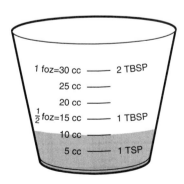

Drug Label Problem #6

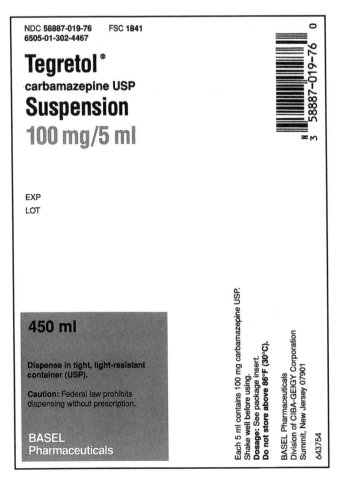

NDC 58887-019-76   FSC 1841
6505-01-302-4467

Tegretol®
carbamazepine USP
Suspension
100 mg/5 ml

EXP
LOT

450 ml

Dispense in tight, light-resistant container (USP).

Caution: Federal law prohibits dispensing without prescription.

BASEL
Pharmaceuticals

Each 5 ml contains 100 mg carbamazepine USP.
Shake well before using.
Dosage: See package insert.
Do not store above 86°F (30°C).

BASEL Pharmaceuticals
Division of CIBA-GEIGY Corporation
Summit, New Jersey 07901

643754

58887-019-76

Figure   4-13. Tegretol®/carbamazepine.
(Courtesy of Basel Pharmaceuticals)

Order: Tegretol 100 mg PO qid for convulsions. How many tsp will you give?

Given quantity   = 100 mg

Wanted quantity = tsp

Dose on hand   = 100 mg/5 mL

Random method:

$$\frac{100 \text{ mg}}{} \bigg| \frac{1 \text{ tsp}}{5 \text{ mL}} \bigg| \frac{5 \text{ mL}}{100 \text{ mg}} \bigg| \frac{1}{} = 1 \text{ tsp}$$

The wanted quantity and the answer to the problem is 1 tsp.

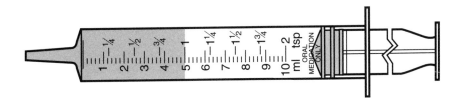

Practice Problems with Liquid Medication

1. Order: phenobarbital gr $\frac{1}{2}$ PO daily for convulsions.

   On hand: 20 mg/5 mL
   How many mL will you give?

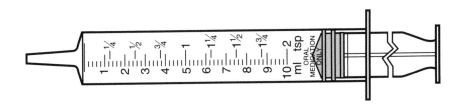

2. Order: Zantac 0.15 g PO bid for ulcers.
   On hand: 15 mg/mL
   How many tsp will you give?

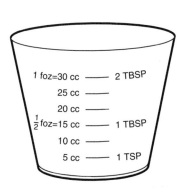

3. Order: Dilaudid 3 mg PO every 3 hour PRN for pain.
   On hand: Dilaudid Liquid 1 mg/mL
   How many mL will you give?

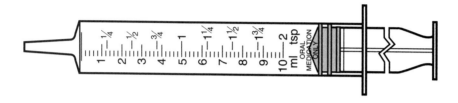

4. Order: lactulose 20 g PO tid for hepatic encephalopathy.
   On hand: lactulose 10 g/15 mL
   How many oz will you give?

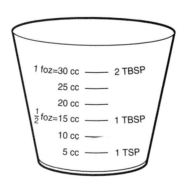

Medications may also be ordered by the physician for the parenteral route of administration, including subcutaneous (SQ), intramuscular (IM), and intravenous (IV). Parenteral medications are sterile solutions obtained from vials or ampules and are administered using a syringe or prefilled syringes. The three syringes most often used include:

1. 3-cc syringe (used for a variety of medications requiring administration of 0.2 to 3 cc).
2. Insulin syringe (used specifically to administer insulin).
3. Tuberculin syringe (used for a variety of medications requiring administration of doses from 0.1 to 1 cc).

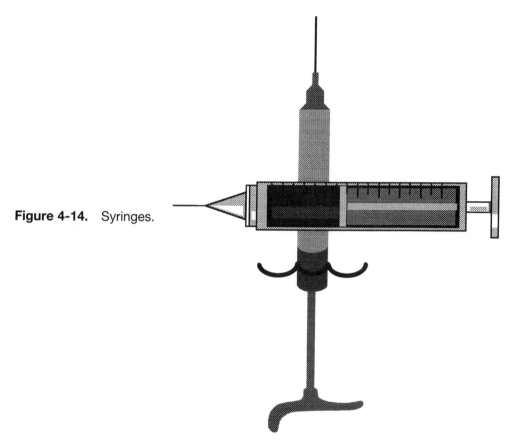

Figure 4-14. Syringes.

Drug Label Problem #7

Figure 4-15. Tigan®/trimethobenzamide HCl. (Courtesy of SmithKline Beecham Pharmaceuticals)

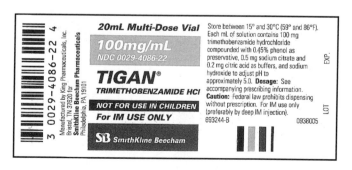

Order: Tigan 100 mg IM qid, for nausea. How many mL will you give?

Given quantity   = 100 mg

Wanted quantity = mL

Dose on hand   = 100 mg/mL

Sequential method:

$$\frac{100 \text{ mg}}{} \left| \frac{\text{mL}}{100 \text{ mg}} \right| \frac{1}{1} = 1 \text{ mL}$$

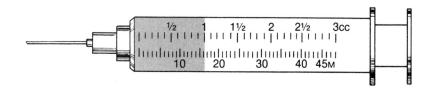

Drug Label Problem #8

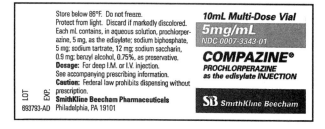

Store below 86°F. Do not freeze.
Protect from light. Discard if markedly discolored.
Each mL contains, in aqueous solution, prochlorper-
azine, 5 mg, as the edisylate; sodium biphosphate,
5 mg; sodium tartrate, 12 mg; sodium saccharin,
0.9 mg; benzyl alcohol, 0.75%, as preservative.
Dosage: For deep I.M. or I.V. injection.
See accompanying prescribing information.
Caution: Federal law prohibits dispensing without
prescription.
SmithKline Beecham Pharmaceuticals
693793-AD Philadelphia, PA 19101
LOT
EXP.

10mL Multi-Dose Vial
5mg/mL
NDC 0007-3343-01
COMPAZINE®
PROCHLORPERAZINE
as the edisylate INJECTION
SB SmithKline Beecham

Figure 4-16. Compazine®/prochloropera-zine. (Courtesy of SmithKline Beecham Pharmaceuticals)

Order: Compazine, 10 mg IM every 4 hour, for psychoses. How many mL will you give?

Given quantity   = 10 mg

Wanted quantity = mL

Dose on hand   = 5 mg/mL

Sequential method:

$$\frac{10 \text{ mg} \left|\text{mL}\right| 10}{\left|5 \text{ mg}\right| 5} = 2 \text{ mL}$$

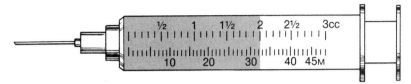

Drug Label Problem #9

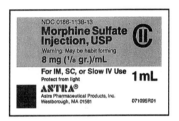

Figure 4-17. Morphine sulfate. (Courtesy of Astra Pharmaceutical Products)

Order: morphine sulfate, $\frac{1}{4}$ gr every 4 hour prn for pain. How many mL will you give?

Given quantity $= \frac{1}{4}$ gr

Wanted quantity $=$ mL

Dose on hand $= 8$ mg/mL or $\frac{1}{8}$ gr/mL

Random method:

$$\frac{\frac{1}{4} \text{ gr} \left|\text{mL}\right| 60 \text{ mg} \left|\frac{1}{4} \times \frac{60}{1}\right| \frac{60}{4} \left| 15 \right.}{\left|8 \text{ mg}\right| 1 \text{ gr} \left| 8 \times 1 \right| 8 \left| 8 \right.} = 1.87 \text{ mL or } 1.8 \text{ mL}$$

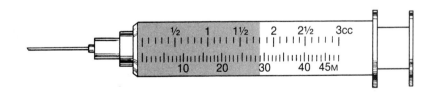

Drug Label Problem #10

Order: NPH Human Insulin, 20 units SQ every AM, for type I diabetes mellitus. How many units will you give?

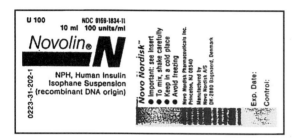

Figure 4-18. Novolin®/NPH human insulin (Courtesy of Novo Nordisk Pharmaceutical)

Sequential method:

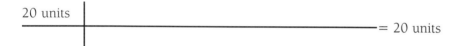

$$\frac{20\ units}{} = 20\ units$$

• • • • • THINKING THROUGH THE PROBLEM

Insulin is given with an insulin syringe that requires no calculation. The number of units of insulin ordered by the physician equals the number of units that the nurse draws up in the insulin syringe.

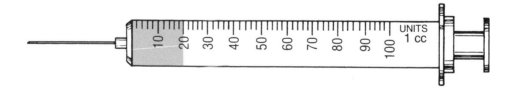

Drug Label Problem #11

Order: Lente human insulin, 45 units SQ every AM, for type I diabetes mellitus. How many units will you give?

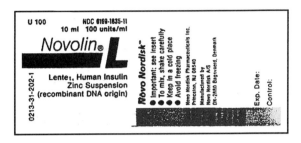

Figure 4-19. Novolin®/Lente human insulin. (Courtesy of Nove Nordisk Pharmaceutical)

Sequential method:

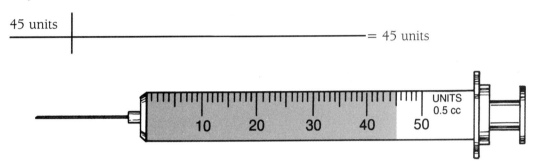

45 units _____= 45 units

Drug Label Problem #12

Order: heparin, 5000 units SQ bid, for prevention of thrombi.
On hand: heparin 10,000 units/mL
How many mL will you give?
Sequential method:

$$\frac{5{,}000 \text{ units}}{} \cdot \frac{\text{mL}}{10{,}000 \text{ units}} \cdot \frac{5}{10} = 0.5 \text{ mL}$$

• • • • • THINKING THROUGH THE PROBLEM

Heparin is administered using a tuberculin syringe because it is calibrated from 0.1 to 1 cc, which allows more accurate administration of medication dosages of less than 1 cc.

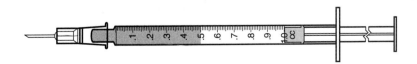

Practice Problems with Parenteral Medications

1. Order: atropine sulfate, 300 mcg IM, for preoperative medication. How many mL will you give?

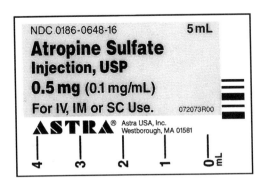

Figure 4-20. Atropine sulfate. (Courtesy of Astra Pharmaceutical Products)

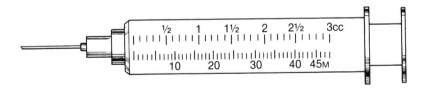

2. Order: hydromorphone, 3 mg IM every 4 hours, for pain. How many mL will you give?

Figure 4-21. Hydromorphone HCl. (Courtesy of Astra Pharmaceutical Products)

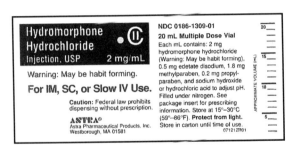

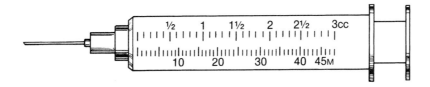

3. Order: meperidine 35 mg IV every hour for pain. How many mL will you give?

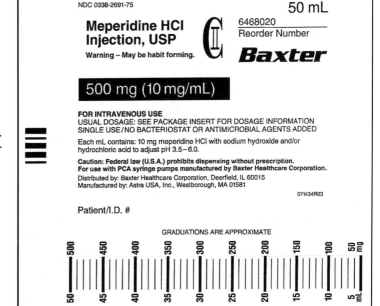

Figure 4-22. Meperidine HCl. (Courtesy of Baxter Pharmaceuticals)

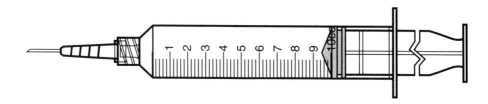

4. Order: regular insulin, 10 units SQ every AM, for type I diabetes mellitus.
   On hand: regular insulin 100 units/mL
   How many units will you give?

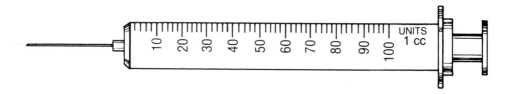

5. Order: heparin, 8000 units SQ bid, for prevention of thrombi.
   On hand: heparin 10,000 units/mL
   How many mL will you give?

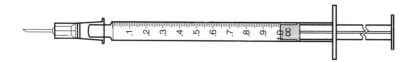

This chapter has assisted the learner to interpret medication orders and drug labels correctly and to accurately calculate one-factor–given quantity to one-factor–wanted quantity medication problems using the sequential or random problem-solving methods of dimensional analysis. To demonstrate your ability to interpret correctly and calculate accurately, complete the following practice problems.

Practice Problems

1. The physician orders Tigan, 0.2 g IM qid, for nausea.
   The dosage of medication on hand is a multiple-dose vial labeled 100 mg/mL.
   How many mL will you give?

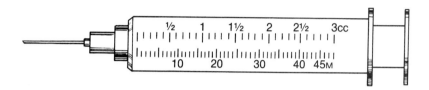

2. A physician orders Thorazine, 50 mg tid, prn for singultus.
   The dose on hand is Thorazine 25 mg tablets.
   How many tablets will you give?

3. Order: Orinase, 1 g PO bid, for type II diabetes mellitus.
   How many tablets will you give?

Figure 4-23. Orinase®/tolbutamide. (Courtesy of the Upjohn Company)

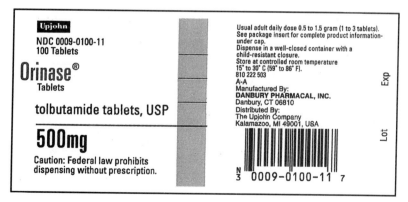

4. Order: Persantine, 50 mg PO qid, for prevention of thromboembolism.
   How many tablets will you give?

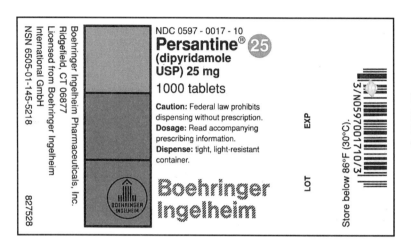

Figure 4-24. Persantine®/dipyridamole. (Courtesy of Boehringer Ingelheim Pharmaceutical)

5. Order: NPH insulin, 56 units SQ, every AM for type I diabetes mellitus.
   On hand: NPH insulin 100 units/mL.
   How many units will you give?

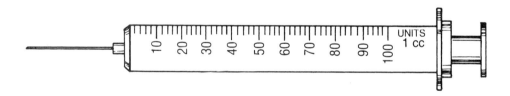

6. Order: heparin, 7500 units SQ bid, for prevention of thrombi.
   On hand: heparin 10,000 units/mL
   How many mL will you give?

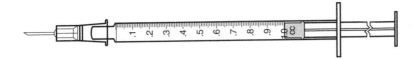

7. Order: Augmentin, 500 mg PO every 8 hours, for infection.
   How many mL will you give?

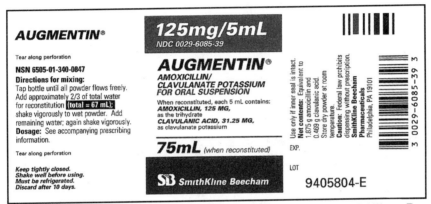

Figure 4-25. Augmentin®/amoxicillin. (Courtesy of SmithKline Beecham Pharmaceuticals)

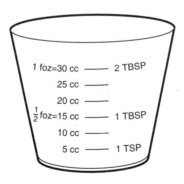

8. Order: Zaroxolyn, 5 mg PO every AM, for hypertension.
   How many tablets will you give?

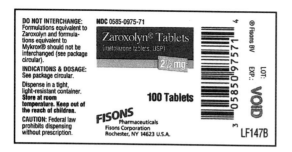

Figure 4-26. Zaroxolyn®/metolazone. (Courtesy of Fisons Pharmaceuticals)

9. Order: Compazine, 10 mg PO bid, for emotional disturbance.
   How many capsules will you give?

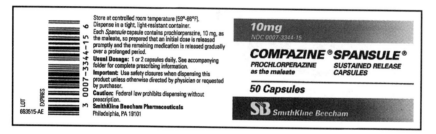

Figure 4-27. Compazine®/ Prochlorperazine. (Courtesy of SmithKline Beecham Pharmaceuticals)

10. Order: meperidine, 50 mg IM, every 3 hours prn for pain.
    On hand: meperidine 100 mg/mL.
    How many mL will you give?

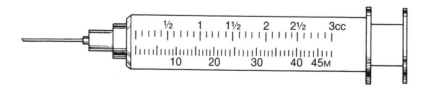

5 Two-Factor Medication Problems

Chapter Objectives

After completing this chapter the learner will be able to

1. Solve two-factor–given quantity to one-factor–wanted quantity medication problems involving a specific amount of medication ordered based on the weight of the patient.

2. Calculate medication problems requiring reconstitution of medications before administration by using information from a nursing drug reference, label, or package insert.

3. Solve two-factor–given quantity to two-factor–wanted quantity medication problems involving a specific amount of fluid to be delivered over a limited amount of time using an intravenous pump delivering milliliters per hour (mL/hr).

4. Solve two-factor–given quantity to two-factor–wanted quantity medication problems involving a specific amount of fluid to be delivered over a limited amount of time using different types of intravenous tubing that deliver drops per minute (gtt/min) based on a specific *drop factor*.

Although medications are ordered by physicians and administered by nurses using the "five rights of medication administration," other factors might need to be considered when administering certain medications or intravenous fluids. The *weight* of the patient often must be factored into a medication problem when determining how much medication can safely be given to an infant or a child or the elderly. The dosage of medication available may be in a powdered form and need *reconstitution* to a liquid form before parenteral or intravenous administration. Also, the length of *time* over which medications or intravenous fluids can be given plays an important role in the safe administration of intravenous therapy.

To be able to calculate a two-factor–given quantity to one-factor– or two-factor–wanted quantity medication problem, it is important to understand all factors that may need to be considered in some medication problems. With use of dimensional analysis, this chapter will assist the learner to accurately calculate medication problems involving the weight of the patient, the reconstitution of medications from powder to liquid form, and the amount of time over which medications or intravenous fluids can be safely administered.

◻ Medication Problems Involving Weight

When using the five steps involved in problem-solving with dimensional analysis, either the *sequential method* or the *random method* can be used to calculate two-factor–given quantity medication problems without difficulty. The **given quantity** (the physician's order) now contains two parts including a **numerator** (dosage of medication) and a **denominator** (the weight of the patient). This type of medication problem is called a *two-factor* medication problem because the *given quantity* now contains two parts (a numerator and a denominator) instead of just one part (a numerator).

Below is an example of the problem-solving method showing placement of basic terms used in dimensional analysis, applied to a two-factor medication problem involving weight.

	Unit Path				
Given Quantity	Conversion Factor For Given Quantity (Numerator)	Conversion Factor For Given Quantity (Denominator)		Conversion Computation	Wanted Quantity
2.5 mg	mL	1 kg	60 lb	$2.5 \times 1 \times 6$	$\dfrac{15}{8.8} = 1.7$ mL
kg	40 mg	2.2 lb		4.22	

Problem Example #1

The physician orders gentamicin 2.5 mg/kg IV (intravenous) every 8 hours for infection. The vial of medication is labeled 40 mg/mL. The child weighs 60 lb. How many milliliters will you give?

Given quantity   = 2.5 mg/kg

Wanted quantity = mL

Dose on hand   = 40 mg/mL

Weight   = 60 lb

• • • • • **THINKING THROUGH THE PROBLEM**

Identify the two-factor–given quantity (the physician's order), which contains two parts including a numerator (2.5 mg) and a denominator (kg). Identify the one-factor–wanted quantity (mL). Establish the unit path from the given quantity to the wanted quantity using equivalents as conversion factors.

Sequential method:

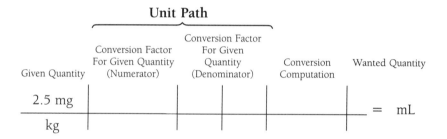

• • • • • **THINKING THROUGH THE PROBLEM**

The two-factor–given quantity has been set up correctly with a numerator (2.5 mg) and a denominator (kg) leading across the unit path to a one-factor–wanted quantity with only a numerator (mL).

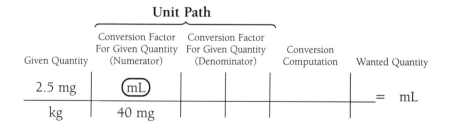

• • • • • THINKING THROUGH THE PROBLEM

The *dose on hand* (40 mg/mL) has been factored into the unit path to cancel out the preceding unwanted unit (mg). The wanted unit (mL) is in the numerator portion of the unit path and correctly corresponds with the one-factor–wanted quantity (mL).

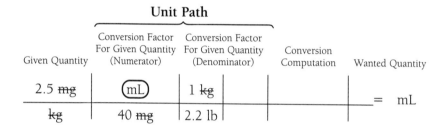

• • • • • THINKING THROUGH THE PROBLEM

A *conversion factor* (1 kg = 2.2 lb) is now factored into the unit path to cancel out the preceding unwanted unit (kg).

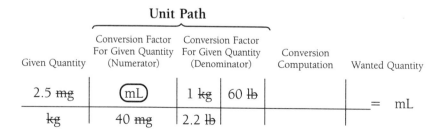

• • • • • THINKING THROUGH THE PROBLEM

The *weight* is finally factored into the unit path to cancel out the preceding unwanted unit (lb) in the denominator portion of the problem. All unwanted units are now canceled from the problem and only the wanted unit (mL) remains in the numerator portion of the unit path and correctly corresponds with the one-factor–wanted quantity (mL). Multiply the numerators, multiply the denominators, and divide the product of the numerators by the product of the denominators to provide the numerical value for the one-factor–wanted quantity.

Unit Path

Given Quantity	Conversion Factor For Given Quantity (Numerator)	Conversion Factor For Given Quantity (Denominator)		Conversion Computation	Wanted Quantity
$\dfrac{2.5 \text{ mg}}{\text{kg}}$	$\dfrac{\text{mL}}{40 \text{ mg}}$	$\dfrac{1 \text{ kg}}{2.2 \text{ lb}}$	60 lb	$\dfrac{2.5 \times 1 \times 6}{4.22}$	$\dfrac{15}{8.8} = 1.7 \text{ mL}$

The *wanted quantity* is 1.7 ml, and is the answer to the problem.
Random method:

$$\frac{2.5 \text{ mg}}{\text{kg}} \bigg| \frac{1 \text{ kg}}{2.2 \text{ lb}} \bigg| 60 \text{ lb} \bigg| \frac{\text{mL}}{40 \text{ mg}} \bigg| \frac{2.5 \times 1 \times 6}{2.2 \times 4} \bigg| \frac{15}{8.8} = 1.7 \text{ mL}$$

• • • • • THINKING THROUGH THE PROBLEM

Dimensional analysis is a problem-solving method that uses critical thinking. When implementing the *random method* of dimensional analysis, the medication problem can be set up in a number of different ways. The focus is on the correct placement of the conversion factors to cancel out all unwanted units. The wanted unit is placed in the numerator portion of the problem to correctly correspond with the wanted quantity.

Practice Problems Involving Weight

1. Order: furosemide 1 mg/kg IV bid for hypercalcemia. The child weighs 45 lb. How many milliliters will you give?

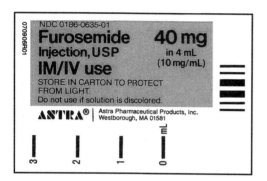

Figure 5-1. Furosemide. (Courtesy of Astra Pharmaceutical Products)

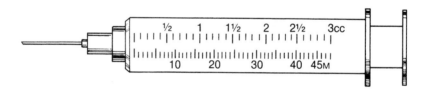

2. Order: atropine sulfate, 0.01 mg/kg IV stat, for bradycardia. The child weighs 20 lb. How many milliliters will you give?

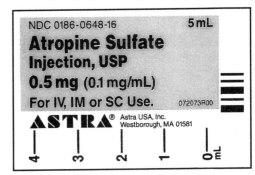

Figure 5-2. Atropine sulfate. (Courtesy of Astra Pharmaceutical Products).

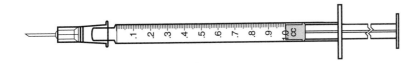

3. Order: phenergan, 0.5 mg/kg IV every 4 hours prn, for nausea. The dose on hand is 25 mg/mL. The child weighs 45 lb. How many milliliters will you give?

4. Order: morphine, 50 mcg/kg IV every 4 hours prn, for pain. The child weighs 75 lb. How many milliliters will you give?

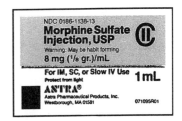

Figure 5-3. Morphine sulfate. (Courtesy of Astra Pharmaceutical Products).

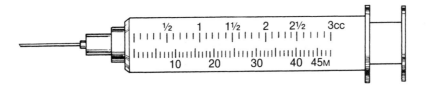

5. Order: Tagamet, 10 mg/kg PO qid, for prophylaxis of duodenal ulcer.
   Supply: Tagamet 300 mg/5 mL
   Child's weight: 70 lb
   How many milliliters will you give?

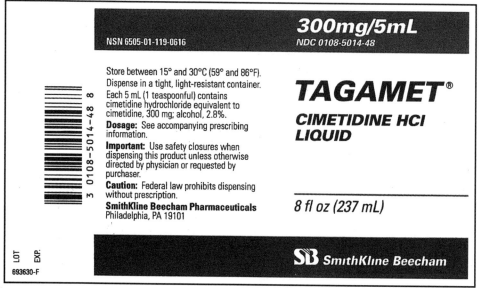

Figure 5-4. Tagamet®/cimetidine HCl. (Courtesy of SmithKline Beecham Pharmaceuticals)

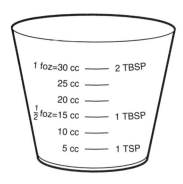

⬭ **Medication Problems Involving Reconstitution**

Some medications in vials are in a powder form and need reconstitution before administration. **Reconstitution** involves adding a specific amount of sterile solution (also called **diluent**) to the vial to change the powder to a liquid form. Information on how much diluent to add to the vial and what dosage of medication per milliliter will result after reconstitution (also called **yield**) can be obtained from a nursing drug reference, label, or package insert.

Problem Example #2

The physician orders Mezlin (mezlocillin), 50 mg/kg every 4 hours IV, for infection. The child weighs 60 lb. The pharmacy sends a vial of medication labeled Mezlin 1 g. The nursing drug reference provides information to reconstitute 1 g of medication with 10 mL of sterile water for injection, 0.9% NaCl, or D5W. How many milliliters will you draw from the vial?

Given quantity   = 50 mg/kg

Wanted quantity = mL

Dose on hand   = 1 g/10 mL (yields 1 g/10 mL)

Weight   = 60 lb

Random method:

Unit Path

Given Quantity	Conversion Factor For Given Quantity (Denominator)	Conversion Factor For Given Quantity (Numerator)		Conversion Computation	Wanted Quantity
$\dfrac{50 \text{ mg}}{\text{kg}}$	$\dfrac{1 \text{ kg}}{2.2 \text{ lb}}$	$\dfrac{60 \text{ lb}}{}$ $\dfrac{10 \text{ (mL)}}{1 \text{ gm}}$	$\dfrac{1 \text{ gm}}{1000 \text{ mg}}$	$\dfrac{5 \times 1 \times 6}{2.2}$	$\dfrac{30}{2.2} = 13.63 \text{ mL}$

The wanted quantity is 13.63 mL or 13.6 mL and is the answer to the problem.

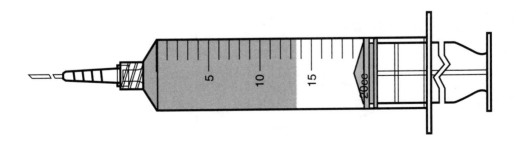

Problem Example #3

Order: Solu-Medrol, 40 mg IV every 4 hours, for inflammation. How many milliliters will you draw from the vial?

Solu-Medrol®

Upjohn

brand of methylprednisolone sodium succinate sterile powder
(methylprednisolone sodium succinate for injection, USP)

For Intravenous or Intramuscular Administration

125 mg Act-O-Vial System (Single-Dose Vial)—Each 2 mL (when mixed) contains methyl-prednisolone sodium succinate equivalent to 125 mg methylprednisolone; also 1.6 mg monobasic sodium phosphate anhydrous; 17.4 mg dibasic sodium phosphate dried; 17.6 mg benzyl alcohol added as preservative.

DOSAGE AND ADMINISTRATION

When high dose therapy is desired, the recommended dose of SOLU-MEDROL Sterile Powder is 30 mg/kg administered intravenously over at least 30 minutes. This dose may be repeated every 4 to 6 hours for 48 hours.

In general, high dose corticosteroid therapy should be continued only until the patient's condition has stabilized; usually not beyond 48 to 72 hours.

Although adverse effects associated with high dose short-term corticoid therapy are uncommon, peptic ulceration may occur. Prophylactic antacid therapy may be indicated.

In other indications initial dosage will vary from 10 to 40 mg of methylprednisolone depending on the clinical problem being treated. The larger doses may be required for short-term management of severe, acute conditions. The initial dose usually should be given intravenously over a period of several minutes. Subsequent doses may be given intravenously or intramuscularly at intervals dictated by the patient's response and clinical condition. Corticoid therapy is an adjunct to, and not replacement for conventional therapy.

Dosage may be reduced for infants and children but should be governed more by the severity of the condition and response of the patient than by age or size. It should not be less than 0.5 mg per kg every 24 hours.

Dosage must be decreased or discontinued gradually when the drug has been administered for more than a few days. If a period of spontaneous remission occurs in a chronic condition, treatment should be discontinued. Routine laboratory studies, such as urinalysis, two-hour postprandial blood sugar, determination of blood pressure and body weight, and a chest X-ray should be made at regular intervals during prolonged therapy. Upper GI X-rays are desirable in patients with an ulcer history or significant dyspepsia.

SOLU-MEDROL may be administered by intravenous or intramuscular injection or by intra-venous infusion, the preferred method for initial emergency use being intravenous injection. To administer by intravenous (or intramuscular) injection, prepare solution as directed. The desired dose may be administered intravenously over a period of several minutes. If desired, the medication may be administered in diluted solutions by adding Water for Injection or other suitable diluent (see below) to the **Act-O-Vial** and withdrawing the indicated dose.

To prepare solutions for intravenous infusion, first prepare the solution for injection as directed. This solution may then be added to indicated amounts of 5% dextrose in water, iso-tonic saline solution or 5% dextrose in isotonic saline solution.

Multiple Sclerosis

In treatment of acute exacerbations of multiple sclerosis, daily doses of 200 mg of pred-nisolone for a week followed by 80 mg every other day for 1 month have been shown to be effective (4 mg of methylprednisolone is equivalent to 5 mg of prednisolone).

DIRECTIONS FOR USING THE ACT-O-VIAL SYSTEM

1. Press down on plastic activator to force diluent into the lower compartment.
2. Gently agitate to effect solution.
3. Remove plastic tab covering center of stopper.
4. Sterilize top of stopper with a suitable germicide.
5. Insert needle **squarely through center** of stopper until tip is just visible. Invert vial and withdraw dose.

STORAGE CONDITIONS

Store unreconstituted product at controlled room temperature 15° to 30° C (59° to 86° F). Store solution at controlled room temperature 15° to 30° C (59° to 86° F). Use solution within 48 hours after mixing.

HOW SUPPLIED

SOLU-MEDROL Sterile Powder is available in the following packages:

40 mg Act-O-Vial System (Single-Dose Vial)	**500 mg** Vial NDC 0009-0758-01
1 mL NDC 0009-0113-12	**500 mg** Vial with Diluent NDC 0009-0887-01
25—1 mL NDC 0009-0113-13	**500 mg Act-O-Vial System (Single-Dose Vial)**
25—1 mL NDC 0009-0113-19	4 mL NDC 0009-0765-02
125 mg Act-O-Vial System (Single-Dose Vial)	1 gram Vial NDC 0009-0698-01
2 mL NDC 0009-0190-09	**1 gram Act-O-Vial System (Single-Dose Vial)**
25—2 mL NDC 0009-0190-10	8 mL NDC 0009-3389-01
25—2 mL NDC 0009-0190-16	**2 gram** Vial NDC 0009-0988-01
	2 gram Vial with Diluent NDC 0009-0796-01

Figure 5-5. Package insert for Solu-Medrol®/methylprednisolone. (Courtesy of the Upjohn Company)

Given quantity   = 40 mg

Wanted quantity = mL

Dose on hand   = 125 mg/2 mL (yield from 2 mL Act-O-Vial)

Sequential method:

$$\frac{40 \ \text{mg}}{} \left| \frac{2 \ \text{(mL)}}{125 \ \text{mg}} \right| \frac{40 \times 2}{125} \left| \frac{80}{125} \right. = 0.64 \ \text{mL or } 0.6 \ \text{mL}$$

The wanted quantity is 0.6 mL and is the answer to the problem.

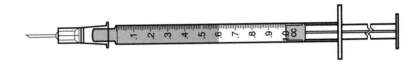

Problem Example #4

Order: Claforan, 50 mg/kg IV every 8 hours, for infection. The infant weighs 12 kg. How many milliliters will you draw from the vial after reconstitution?
Supply: Claforan 1 g/10 mL

719000-2/95

Claforan®

**Sterile (sterile cefotaxime sodium)
and
Injection (cefotaxime sodium injection)**

**HOECHST-ROUSSEL
Pharmaceuticals Incorporated
Somerville, NJ 08876-1258**

REG TM HOECHST AG

Neonates, Infants, and Children
The following dosage schedule is recommended:

Neonates (birth to 1 month):
0-1 week of age   50 mg/kg per dose every 12 hours IV
1-4 weeks of age   50 mg/kg per dose every 8 hours IV
It is not necessary to differentiate between premature and normal-gestational age infants.
Infants and Children (1 month to 12 years): For body weights less than 50 kg, the recommended daily dose is 50 to 180 mg/kg
IM or IV body weight divided into four to six equal doses. The higher dosages should be used for more severe or serious infections,
including meningitis. For body weights 50 kg or more, the usual adult dosage should be used; the maximum daily dosage should not
exceed 12 grams.

Figure 5-6. Claforan®/cefotaxime sodium package insert. (Courtesy of Hoechst-Roussel Pharmaceuticals)

Given quantity   = 50 mg/kg

Wanted quantity = mL

Dose on hand   = 1 g/10 mL

Weight   = 12 kg

Random method:

$$\frac{50\ \text{mg}}{\text{kg}}\left|\frac{10\ \text{(mL)}}{1\ \text{g}}\right|\frac{1\ \text{g}}{1000\ \text{mg}}\left|\frac{12\ \text{kg}}{}\right|\frac{5 \times 1 \times 12}{1 \times 10}\left|\frac{60}{10}\right. = 6\ \text{mL}$$

The wanted quantity is 6 mL and is the answer to the problem.

• • • • • THINKING THROUGH THE PROBLEM

The package inserts provide information on how to reconstitute the medication for intravenous use: Reconstitute vials with at least 10 mL of sterile water for injection.

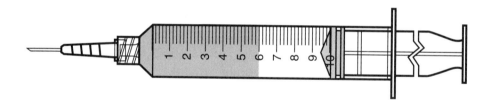

• • • • • THINKING THROUGH THE PROBLEM

A nursing drug reference, label, or package insert will provide information on how much and what type of *diluent* to use to reconstitute a drug as well as what would be the *yield* or reconstitution. The five problem-solving steps of dimensional analysis remain applicable with any reconstitution medication problem.

Practice Problems Involving Reconstitution

1. Order: Ancef, 500 mg IV every 8 hours, for infection. How many milliliters will you draw out of the vial after reconstitution?
   (Ancef is reconstituted using 50 mL Sodium Chloride)

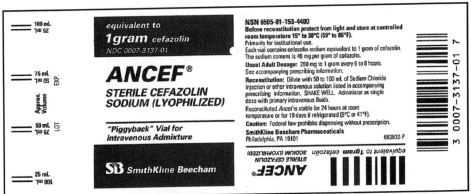

Figure 5-7. Ancef®/cefazolin. (Courtesy of SmithKline Beecham Pharmaceuticals)

2. Order: Primaxin, 250 mg IV every 6 hours, for infection
   Supply: Primaxin vial labeled 500 mg. Reconstitute with 10 mL of compatible diluent and shake well. How many milliliters will you draw from the vial after reconstitution?

3. Order: Unasyn (ampicillin), 50 mg/kg IV every 4 hours, for infection
   Supply: Unasyn 1.5-g vial
   Nursing drug reference: Reconstitute each Unasyn 1.5-g vial with 4 mL of sterile water to yield 375 mg/mL
   The child weighs 40 kg
   How many milliliters will you draw from the vial after reconstitution?

4. Order: erythromycin, 750 mg IV every 6 hours, for infection
   Supply: erythromycin 1-g vial labeled: Reconstitute with 20 mL of sterile water for
   injection.
   How many milliliters will you draw from the vial after reconstitution?

5. Order: Fortaz, 30 mg/kg IV every 8 hours, for infection
   Supply: Fortaz 500-mg vial labeled: Reconstitute with 5 mL of sterile water for injection
   The child weighs 65 lb
   How many milliliters will you draw from the vial after reconstitution?

☐ Medication Problems Involving Intravenous Pumps

Intravenous medications are administered by drawing a specific amount of medication from a vial or ampule and inserting that medication into an existing intravenous line. All intravenous medications must be given with specific thought to exactly how much *time* it should take to administer the medication. Information regarding time may be obtained from a nursing drug reference, label, or package insert, or may be specifically ordered by the physician.

Although IV medications can be administered IV push, often the time involved requires the use of an intravenous pump (IV pump). All IV pumps deliver milliliters per hour (mL/hr or cc/hr) but may vary in operational capacity or size.

Below is an example of the dimensional analysis problem-solving method with basic terms applied to a medication problem involving an IV pump.

Unit Path

Given Quantity	Conversion Factor For Given Quantity (Numerator)	Conversion Computation	Wanted Quantity
$\dfrac{1500 \text{ Units}}{\text{hr}}$	$\dfrac{250 \text{ mL}}{25000 \text{ Units}}$	$\dfrac{15}{\text{hr}}$	$= \quad 15 \text{ mL}$

Problem Example #5

The physician orders heparin, 1500 units/hr IV. The pharmacy sends an IV bag labeled: Heparin 25,000 units in 250 mL of D5W. Calculate the IV pump setting for milliliters per hour.

Given quantity   = 1500 units/hr

Wanted quantity = mL/hr

Dose on hand   = 25,000 units/250 mL

Begin by identifying the *given quantity* and establish the unit path to the *wanted quantity*.

Sequential method:

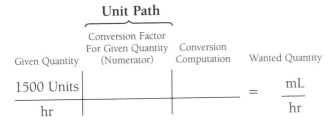

• • • • • THINKING THROUGH THE PROBLEM

The two-factor–given quantity (the physician's order) contains two parts including a **numerator** (the dosage of medication) and a **denominator** (time). The wanted quantity (the answer to the problem) also contains two parts including a numerator (mL) and a denominator (time). This is called a two-factor–given quantity to a two-factor–wanted quantity medication problem. The denominator portion of the given quantity (hr) corresponds with the denominator portion of the wanted quantity (hr); therefore, only the numerator portion of the given quantity (units) needs to be canceled from the problem.

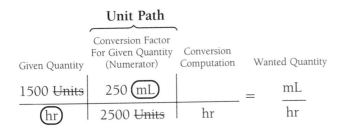

••••• THINKING THROUGH THE PROBLEM

After factoring the dose on hand into the unit path, the unwanted unit (units) is canceled from the problem and the wanted unit (mL) remains in the numerator portion of the problem to correspond with the wanted quantity. The same number of zeros and the same number values are canceled from the numerator and denominator portions of the problem leaving 15 mL/hr as the wanted quantity and the answer to the problem.

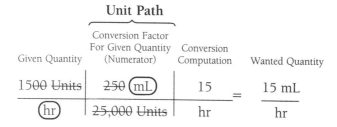

Unit Path

Conversion Factor
For Given Quantity   Conversion
Given Quantity   (Numerator)   Computation   Wanted Quantity

$$\frac{1500 \ \text{Units}}{\text{hr}} \left| \frac{250 \ \text{mL}}{25,000 \ \text{Units}} \right| \frac{15}{\text{hr}} = \frac{15 \ \text{mL}}{\text{hr}}$$

Problem Example #6

The physician orders 500 mL of 0.45% NS with 20 mEq of KCl to infuse over 8 hours. Calculate the number of milliliters per hour to set the IV pump.

Given quantity = 500 mL/8 hr

Wanted quantity = mL/hr

Sequential method:

$$\frac{500 \ \text{mL}}{8 \ \text{hr}} \left| \frac{500}{8} \right. = \frac{62.5 \ \text{mL}}{} \ \text{or} \ \frac{63 \ \text{mL}}{\text{hr}}$$

The wanted quantity is 63 mL/hr and is the answer to the problem.

• • • • • THINKING THROUGH THE PROBLEM

In this problem the two factors needed for the wanted quantity are already identified in the given quantity and, therefore, require no additional conversions added to the unit path. The 20 mEq of KCl added to the IV bag is included as part of the 500 mL and is additional information for the nurse, but not part of the calculation.

Problem Example #7

The physician orders aminophylline 44 mg/hr IV. The pharmacy sends an IV bag labeled: Aminophylline 1 g/250 mL NS. Calculate the milliliters per hour to set the IV pump?

Given quantity   = 44 mg/hr

Wanted quantity = mL/hr

Dose on hand   = 1 g/250 mL

Random method:

$$\frac{44\ \text{mg}}{\text{hr}} \left| \frac{250\ \text{mL}}{1\ \text{g}} \right| \frac{1\ \text{g}}{1000\ \text{mg}} \left| \frac{44 \times 25}{100} \right| \frac{1100}{100} = \frac{11\ \text{mL}}{\text{hr}}$$

The wanted quantity is 11 mL/hr and is the answer to the problem.

• • • • • THINKING THROUGH THE PROBLEM

The given quantity has been identified as what the physician orders, but also can be information that the nurse has obtained. The nurse may know that the IV pump is set to deliver 11 mL/hr, but wants to know if the dosage of medication the patient is receiving is within a safe dosage range.

Problem Example #8

The nurse checks the IV pump and documents that the pump is set at and delivering 11 mL/hr and that the IV bag hanging is labeled: Aminophylline 1 g/250 mL. How many milligrams per hour is the patient receiving?

Given quantity = 11 mL/hr

Wanted quantity = mg/hr

Dose on hand   = 1 g/250 mL

Sequential method:

$$\frac{11 \text{ mL}}{\text{hr}} \left|\right. = \frac{\text{mg}}{\text{hr}}$$

• • • • • THINKING THROUGH THE PROBLEM

The given quantity is now identified as the information that the nurse has obtained and the wanted quantity is what the nurse would like to know.

$$\frac{11 \text{ mL}}{\text{hr}} \left| \frac{1 \text{ g}}{250 \text{ mL}} \right. = \frac{\text{mg}}{\text{hr}}$$

• • • • • THINKING THROUGH THE PROBLEM

The dose on hand is factored into the unit path and allows the unwanted unit (mL) to be canceled from the problem.

$$\frac{11 \text{ mL}}{\text{hr}} \left| \frac{1 \text{ g}}{250 \text{ mL}} \right| \frac{1000 \text{ mg}}{1 \text{ g}} \left| \frac{11 \times 100}{25} \right| \frac{1100}{25} = \frac{44 \text{ mg}}{\text{hr}}$$

• • • • • THINKING THROUGH THE PROBLEM

By using the five steps of dimensional analysis, a variety of medication problems can be solved. Dimensional analysis is a critical-thinking method that allows calculation of problems by identifying the given quantity (the physician's order or what the nurse knows) and establishing a unit path to the wanted quantity using the sequential method or the random method to solve one-factor or two-factor medication problems.

Practice Problems Involving Intravenous Pumps

1. Order: heparin 1800 units/hr IV
   Supply: heparin 25,000 units/250 mL D5W
   Calculate milliliter per hour to set the IV pump?

2. Order: aminophylline 35 mg/hr IV
   Supply: aminophylline 1 g/250 mL NS
   Calculate milliliters per hour to set the IV pump?

3. Information obtained by the nurse: heparin 25,000 units in 250 mL D5W is infusing at 30 mL/hr.
   How many units per hour is the patient receiving?

4. Information obtained by the nurse: aminophylline 1 g/250 mL NS is infusing at 15 mL/hr.
   How many milligrams per hour is the patient receiving?

5. Order: heparin 900 units/hr IV
   Supply: heparin 25,000 units/500 mL D5W
   Calculate milliliters per hour to set the IV pump?

◯ Medication Problems Involving Drop Factors

Although intravenous pumps are used whenver possible, there are situations (no IV pumps available) and circumstances (outpatient or home-care) that arise when IV pumps are not available and IV fluids or medications might be administered using gravity flow. **Gravity flow** involves calculating the drops per minute (gtt/min) required to infuse IV fluids or medications. When IV fluids or medications are administered using gravity flow it is important to know the drop factor for the IV tubing that is being used. **Drop factor** is the drops per milliliter (gtt/mL) that the IV tubing will produce. There are two types of IV tubing available for gravity flow. *Macro*tubing delivers a large drop and is available in 10 gtt/mL, 15 gtt/mL, and 20 gtt/mL (Table 5-1); and *micro*tubing delivers a small drop and is available in 60 gtt/mL.

Regardless of the IV tubing used, the five steps can be used and the problem can be solved by dimensional analysis as the problem-solving method. Below is an example of a medication problem involving drop factors using the dimensional analysis method, showing basic dimensional analysis terms.

Unit Path

Given Quantity	Conversion Factor For Given Quantity (Numerator)	Conversion Computation		Wanted Quantity
$\dfrac{250 \text{ mL}}{30 \text{ min}}$	$\dfrac{10 \text{ gtt}}{\text{mL}}$	$\dfrac{250 \times 1}{3}$	$\dfrac{250}{3} =$	$\dfrac{83.3 \text{ gtt}}{\text{min}}$

Problem Example #9

The physician orders 250 mL of normal saline to infuse in 30 minutes. The drop factor listed on the IV tubing box is 10 gtt/mL. Calculate the number of drops per minute required to infuse the IV bolus.

Given quantity   = 250 mL/30 min

Wanted quantity = gtt/min

Drop factor   = 10 gtt/mL

• •

Table 5-1. Examples of Different Macrodrip Factors	
Manufacturer	**Drops per Milliliter (gtt/mL)**
Travenol	10
Abbott	15
McGaw	15
Cutter	20

• • • • • **THINKING THROUGH THE PROBLEM**

The given quantity and the wanted quantity both include two factors; therefore, this is a two-factor–given quantity to a two-factor–wanted quantity medication problem. Begin by identifying the given quantity and establish a unit path to the wanted quantity.

Sequential method:

Unit Path

Conversion Factor
For Given Quantity   Conversion
Given Quantity   (Numerator)   Computation   Wanted Quantity

$$\frac{250 \text{ mL}}{30 \text{ min}} \Bigg| \quad \Bigg| \quad = \frac{\text{gtt}}{\text{min}}$$

• • • • • **THINKING THROUGH THE PROBLEM**

The denominators of the given quantity and the wanted quantity are the same (min). The numerator in the given quantity (mL) is an unwanted unit and needs to be canceled from the unit path.

Unit Path

Conversion Factor
For Given Quantity   Conversion
Given Quantity   (Numerator)   Computation   Wanted Quantity

$$\frac{250 \text{ mL}}{30 \text{ min}} \Bigg| \frac{10 \text{ gtt}}{\text{mL}} \Bigg| \quad = \frac{83.3 \text{ gtt}}{\text{min}}$$

• • • • • THINKING THROUGH THE PROBLEM

When the drop factor is factored into the unit path, the unwanted unit (mL) is canceled from the problem and the wanted unit (gtt) is correctly placed in the numerator portion of problem to correspond with the wanted quantity.

Unit Path

Given Quantity	Conversion Factor For Given Quantity (Numerator)	Conversion Computation		Wanted Quantity
250 ~~mL~~	10 (gtt)	250 × 1	250	= 83.3 gtt
30 (min)	~~mL~~	3	3	min

• • • • • THINKING THROUGH THE PROBLEM

After the unwanted units are canceled from the problem, cancel the same number of zeros from the numerator and denominator portions of the problem, multiply the numerators, multiply the denominators, and divide the product of the numerators by the product of the denominators to provide the numerical value for the wanted quantity: 83 gtt/min is the wanted quantity and the answer to the problem.

Problem Example #10

The physician orders 1000 mL of D5W and 0.45% NS to infuse over 8 hours. The drop factor is 20 gtt/mL. Calculate the number of drops per minute required to infuse the IV volume.

Given quantity   = 1000 mL/8 hr

Wanted quantity = gtt/min

Drop factor   = 20 gtt/mL

Sequential method:

$$\frac{1000 \text{ mL}}{8 \text{ hr}} \left| \frac{20 \text{ gtt}}{\text{mL}} \right. = \frac{\text{gtt}}{\text{min}}$$

• • • • • **THINKING THROUGH THE PROBLEM**

The unwanted unit (mL) is canceled from the problem and the wanted unit (gtt) is correctly placed in the numerator portion of the problem. Another unwanted unit (hr) needs to be canceled from the unit path.

$$\frac{1000 \text{ mL}}{8 \text{ hr}} \left| \frac{20 \text{ (gtt)}}{\text{mL}} \right| \frac{1 \text{ hr}}{60 \text{ (min)}} = \frac{\text{gtt}}{\text{min}}$$

• • • • • **THINKING THROUGH THE PROBLEM**

The conversion factor (1 hr = 60 min) has been factored into the problem to allow the unwanted unit (hr) to be canceled from the unit path and the wanted unit (min) is correctly placed in the denominator portion of the problem.

$$\frac{1000 \text{ mL}}{8 \text{ hr}} \left| \frac{20 \text{ (gtt)}}{\text{mL}} \right| \frac{1 \text{ hr}}{60 \text{ (min)}} \left| \frac{1000 \times 2 \times 1}{8 \times 6} \right. \frac{2000}{48} = \frac{41.66 \text{ gtt}}{\text{min}}$$

$$41.66 \frac{\text{gtt}}{\text{min}} \quad \text{or} \quad 42 \frac{\text{gtt}}{\text{min}}$$

The wanted quantity is 42 gtt/min and is the answer to the problem.

• • • • • **THINKING THROUGH THE PROBLEM**

In some situations (home-care) it may be important for the nurse to know exactly how long a specific amount of IV fluid will take to infuse. The physician may order a limited amount of IV fluid to infuse at a specific number of drops per minute (gtt/min).

Problem Example #11

The physician orders 1000 mL of D5W. The drop factor is 10 gtt/mL. The infusion is dripping at 21 gtt/min. How many hours will it take for the IV to infuse?

Given quantity   = 1000 mL

Wanted quantity = hr

Drop factor   = 10 gtt/mL

$$\frac{1000 \text{ mL}}{} = \text{hr}$$

• • • • • **THINKING THROUGH THE PROBLEM**

The given quantity and the wanted quantity have been identified and are both in the numerator portion of the problem; therefore, this is a one-factor–given quantity to a one-factor–wanted quantity medication problem.

$$\frac{1000 \text{ mL}}{} \left| \frac{10 \text{ gtt}}{\text{mL}} \right. = \text{hr}$$

• • • • • **THINKING THROUGH THE PROBLEM**

The drop factor (10 gtt/ml) has been factored into the problem using the sequential method to cancel the unwanted unit (mL) from the unit path.

$$\frac{1000 \text{ mL} \quad | \quad 10 \text{ gtt} \quad | \quad \text{min}}{| \quad \text{mL} \quad | \quad 21 \text{ gtt}} = \text{hr}$$

• • • • • **THINKING THROUGH THE PROBLEM**

The infusing rate of 21 gtt/min has now been factored into the problem to cancel the unwanted unit (gtt) from the unit path.

$$\frac{1000 \text{ mL} | 10 \text{ gtt} | \text{min} | 1 \, (\text{hr})}{| \text{mL} | 21 \text{ gtt} | 60 \text{ min}} = \text{hr}$$

• • • • • **THINKING THROUGH THE PROBLEM**

The conversion factor (1 hr = 60 min) has been factored into the problem to cancel the unwanted unit (min) from the unit path. The wanted unit (hr) remains in the numerator portion of the problem which correctly corresponds with the wanted quantity.

$$\frac{1000 \text{ mL} | 10 \text{ gtt} | \text{min} | 1 \, (\text{hr}) | 1000 \times 1 \times 1 | 1000}{| \text{mL} | 21 \text{ gtt} | 60 \text{ min} | \quad 21 \times 6 \quad | 126} = 7.93 \text{ hr or } 8 \text{ hr}$$

• • • • • **THINKING THROUGH THE PROBLEM**

The wanted quantity is 8 hours and is the answer to the problem. It is safe nursing practice to monitor an infusing IV every 2 hours to make sure it is infusing without difficulty and on time. It may be necessary to hang the next IV after $7\frac{1}{2}$ hours (before the estimated completion time) to keep the IV from running dry.

Practice Problems Involving Drop Factors

1. Order: 800 mL D5W to infuse in 8 hr
   Drop factor: 15 gtt/mL
   Calculate the number of drops per minute

2. Order: Infuse 250 mL NS
   Drop factor: 15 gtt/mL
   Infusion rate: 60 gtt/min
   Calculate the hours to infuse.

3. Order: 150 mL over 60 min
   Drop factor: 10 gtt/mL
   Calculate the number of drops per minute.

4. Order: 1000 mL D5W/0.9% NS
   Drop factor: 15 gtt/mL
   Infusion rate: 50 gtt/min
   Calculate the number of hours to infuse.

5. Order: 500 mL over 4 hr
   Drop factor: 15 gtt/mL
   Calculate the number of drops per minute.

◯ Medication Problems Involving Intermittent Infusion

Intravenous medications can be delivered over a specific amount of time by *intermittent infusion*. When medications are delivered by intermittent infusion, they require the use of an infusion pump. Some medications must be reconstituted and further diluted in a specific type and amount of IV fluid and delivered over a limited time. Other medications do not need to be reconstituted, but must be further diluted in a specific type and amount of IV fluid and delivered over a limited time.

Problem Example #12

The physician ordered erythromycin, 500 mg IV every 6 hr for infection. The pharmacy sends a vial labeled: Erythromycin 1 g. The nursing drug reference provides information to reconstitute 1 g of erythromycin with 20 mL of sterile water and further dilute in 250 mL of 0.9% NS and to infuse over 1 hour.
How many milliliters will you draw from the vial after reconstitution?
Calculate the milliliters per hour to set the IV pump.

• • • • • THINKING THROUGH THE PROBLEM

> This order really contains two problems. The first problem involves deciding how many milliliters to draw from the vial after reconstitution, and the second problem involves how many milliliters per hour to set the IV pump. Calculate each part of the problem using dimensional analysis as a problem-solving method.

How many milliliters will you draw from the vial after reconstitution?

Given quantity = 500 mg

Wanted quantity = mL

Dose on hand = 1 g/20 mL

Random method:

$$\frac{500 \text{ mg}}{} \frac{20 \text{ mL}}{1 \text{ g}} \frac{1 \text{ g}}{1000 \text{ mg}} \frac{5 \times 2}{1} \frac{10}{1} = 10 \text{ mL}$$

• • • • • THINKING THROUGH THE PROBLEM

The wanted quantity is 10 mL, and is the amount that will need to be drawn from the vial and added to the 250 mL of 0.9% NS. After adding the 10 mL to the IV bag, the IV bag will now contain 260 mL.

Calculate milliliter per hour to set the IV pump.

Given quantity   = 260 mL/1 hr

Wanted quantity = mL/hr

Sequential method:

$$\frac{260 \text{ mL}}{1 \text{ hr}} \ \Big| \ \frac{260}{1} = \frac{260 \text{ mL}}{\text{hr}}$$

The IV pump is set at 260 mL/hr to infuse the 500 mg of erythromycin ordered by the physician.
  If an IV pump was unavailable, the infusion could be delivered by gravity using IV tubing with a drop factor of 10 gtt/mL.
  Calculate the drops per minute required to infuse the IV volume.

Given quantity   = 260 mL/1 hr

Wanted quantity = gtt/min

Drop factor   = 10 gtt/mL

Sequential method:

$$\frac{260 \text{ mL}}{1 \text{ hr}} \ \Big| \ \frac{10 \text{ gtt}}{\text{mL}} \ \Big| \ \frac{1 \text{ hr}}{60 \text{ min}} \ \Big| \ \frac{260 \times 1 \times 1}{6} \ \Big| \ \frac{260}{6} = \frac{43.3 \text{ or } 43 \text{ gtt}}{\text{min}}$$

Practice Problems Involving Intermittent Infusion

1. Order: ampicillin, 250 mg IV every 4 hr, for infection
   Supply: ampicillin 1-g vial
   Nursing drug reference: Reconstitute with 10 mL of 0.9% NS and further dilute in 50 mL NS. Infuse over 15 min.

How many milliliters will you draw from the vial after reconstitution?
Calculate milliliters per hour to set the IV pump.
Calculate drops per minute with a drop factor of 10 gtt/mL.

2. Order: clindamycin, 0.3 g IV every 6 hr, for infection
   Supply: clindamycin 600 mg/4-mL vial
   Nursing drug reference: Dilute with 50 mL 0.9% NS and infuse over 15 min.
   How many milliliters will you draw from the vial?
   Calculate milliliters per hour to set the IV pump.
   Calculate drops per minute with a drop factor of 15 gtt/mL.

3. Order: Mezlin, 3 g IV every 4 hr, for infection
   Supply: Mezlin 4-g vial
   Nursing drug reference: Reconstitute each 1-g vial with 10 mL of 0.9% NS and further
   dilute in 100 mL 0.9% NS to infuse over 1 h.
   How many milliliters will you draw from the vial after reconstitution?
   Calculate the milliliters per hour to set the IV pump.
   Calculate the drops per minute with a drop factor of 20 gtt/mL.

4. Order: Unasyn, 1000 mg IV every 6 hr, for infection
   Supply: Unasyn 1.5-g vial
   Nursing drug reference: Reconstitute with 4 mL of 0.9% NS and further dilute with 100
   mL NS to infuse over 1 hr.
   How many milliliters will you draw from the vial after reconstitution?
   Calculate the milliliters per hour to set the IV pump.
   Calculate the drops per minute with a drop factor of 20 gtt/mL.

5. Order: Zantac, 50 mg IV every 6 hr, for ulcers
   Supply: Zantac 25-mg/mL vial
   Nursing drug reference: Dilute with 50 mL 0.9% NS to infuse over 30 min.
   How many milliliters will you draw from the vial?
   Calculate the milliliters per hour to set the IV pump.
   Calculate the drops per minute with a drop factor of 10 gtt/mL.

This chapter has assisted the learner to calculate two-factor medication problems involving the weight of the patient, reconstitution of medications, and the amount of time over which medications and intravenous fluids can be safely administered using the sequential or random method of dimensional analysis. To demonstrate your ability to calculate medication problems accurately, complete the following practice problems.

Practice Problems

1. Order: verapamil, 0.2 mg/kg IV, for arrhythmia
   Supply: verapamil (Isoptin) 5 mg/2 mL
   Child's weight: 10 lb
   How many milliliters will you give?

2. Order: Tylenol Elixir, 10 mg/kg every 4 hr prn, for fever
   Supply: Tylenol Elixir 160 mg/5 mL
   Child's weight: 8 kg
   How many milliliters will you give?

3. Order: Fortaz, 1.25 g IV every 8 hr, for infection
   Supply: Fortaz 2-g vial
   Nursing drug reference: Dilute each 2 g with 10 mL sterile water for injection.
   How many milliliters will you draw from the vial after reconstitution?

4. Order: Unasyn, 750 mg IV every 8 hr, for infection
   Supply: Unasyn 1.5-g vial
   Nursing drug reference: Reconstitute with 4 mL of sterile water for injection.
   How many milliliters will you draw from the vial after reconstitution?

5. Order: heparin, 700 units/hr, for anticoagulation
   Supply: heparin 25,000 units/250 mL NS
   At how many milliliters per hour will you set the IV pump?

6. Information obtained by the nurse: Zantac 150 mg in 250 mL NS is infusing at 11 mL/hr.
   How many milligrams per hour is the patient receiving?

7. Order: 1000 mL D5W/0.9% NS to infuse over 8 hr
   Drop factor: 20 gtt/mL
   Calculate the number of drops per minute.

8. Order: infuse 750 mL NS
   Drop factor: 15 gtt/mL
   Infusion rate: 18 gtt/min
   Calculate the number of hours to infuse.

9. Order: vancomycin, 10 mg/kg IV every 8 hr, for infection
   Supply: vancomycin 500-mg vial
   Infant's weight: 20 lb
   Nursing drug reference: Dilute each 500 mg vial with 10 mL of sterile water for injection and further dilute in 100 mL of 0.9% NS to infuse over 1 hr.
   How many milliliters will you draw from the vial after reconstitution?
   Calculate milliliters per hour to set the IV pump.
   Calculate drops per minute with a drop factor of 10 gtt/mL.

10. Order: acyclovir, 355 mg IV every 8 hr, for herpes
    Supply: acyclovir 500-mg vial
    Nursing drug reference: Reconstitute each 500 mg with 10 mL of sterile water for injection and further dilute in 100 mL NS to infuse over 1 hr
    How many milliliters will you draw from the vial after reconstitution?
    Calculate the milliliters per hour to set the IV pump.
    Calculate the drops per minute with a drop factor of 20 gtt/mL.

6

Three-Factor Medication Problems

Chapter Objectives

After completing this chapter the learner will be able to:

1. Calculate three-factor–given quantity to one-factor–two-factor–, or three-factor–wanted quantity medication problems involving a specific amount of medication or intravenous fluid based on the weight of the patient and the time required for safe administration.

2. Calculate medication problems requiring reconstitution or preparation of medications before administration using information from a nursing drug reference, label, or package insert.

When medications are ordered by physicians for infants and children, the *dosage* of medication (g, mg, mcg, gr) based upon the *weight* of the child must be considered as well as how much medication the child can receive per *dose* or *day*. Although the physician orders the medications, the nurse must be aware of the safe dosage range for administration of medications to infants and children, as well as for adults.

When medications are ordered by physicians for critically ill patients, the patients must be closely monitored by the nurse for effectiveness of the medications. Often the medications or intravenous fluids must be *titrated* for effectiveness, with an increase or decrease in the dosage based on the patient's response to the medications. Factors involved in the safe administration of medications or intravenous fluids for the critically ill patient include the *dosage* of medication based on the combined factors of the *weight* of the patient and the *time* required for administration. The medication may need reconstitution or preparation by the nurse for immediate administration in a critical situation. The weight of the patient also may need to be obtained daily to ensure accurate correlation with the dosage of medication ordered.

To be able to calculate three-factor–given quantity to one-factor–, two-factor–, or three-factor–wanted quantity medication problem, it is necessary to understand all of the components of the medication order and to be able to calculate medication problems in a critical situation. This chapter will assist the learner to accurately calculate medication problems involving the dosage of medication based upon the weight of the patient and the time required for safe administration using dimensional analysis as a problem-solving method.

○ Medication Problems Involving Dosage, Weight, and Time

By using the five problem-solving steps, three-factor–given quantity medication problems can be solved implementing the sequential method or the random method of dimensional analysis. The *given quantity* or the physician's order now contains three parts, including a **numerator** (the dosage of medication ordered) and two **denominators** (the *weight* of the patient and the *time* required for safe administration).

Below is an example of this problem-solving method showing placement of basic dimensional analysis terms applied to a three-factor medication problem.

Unit Path

Given Quantity	Conversion Factor For Given Quantity (Numerator)	Conversion Factor For Given Quantity (Denominator)	Conversion Computation	Wanted Quantity
$\dfrac{30 \text{ mg}}{\text{kg day}}$	$\dfrac{5 \text{ mL}}{300 \text{ mg}}$	22 kg	$\dfrac{3 \times 5 \times 22}{30} \Big| \dfrac{330}{30} =$	$\dfrac{11 \text{ mL}}{\text{day}}$

Problem Example #1

The physician orders Tagamet for gastrointestinal ulcers, 30 mg/kg/day PO, in four divided doses for a child weighing 22 kg. The dose on hand is Tagamet 300 mg/5 mL. How many milliliters per day will the child receive?

Given quantity   = 30 mg/kg/day

Wanted quantity = mL/day

Dose on hand   = 300 mg/5 mL

Weight   = 22 kg

• • • • • THINKING THROUGH THE PROBLEM

Identify the three-factor–given quantity (the physician's order) which contains three parts including a *numerator* (30 mg) and two *denominators* (kg/day). Establish the unit path from the *given quantity* (30 mg/kg/day) to the *two-factor–wanted quantity* (mL/day) using the sequential method of dimensional analysis and the necessary conversion factors.

Sequential method:

$$\frac{30 \text{ mg}}{\text{kg/day}} \quad\bigg| \rule{8cm}{0pt} = \frac{\text{mL}}{\text{day}}$$

• • • • • THINKING THROUGH THE PROBLEM

The three-factor–given quantity has been set up correctly with a numerator (30 mg) and two denominators (kg/day) leading across the unit path to a two-factor–wanted quantity, with a numerator (mL) and a denominator (day). The conversion factors can now be factored into the unit path to allow cancellation of unwanted units.

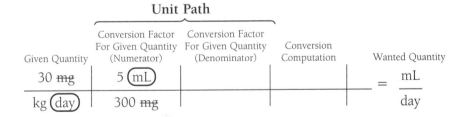

• • • • • THINKING THROUGH THE PROBLEM

The *dose on hand* (300 mg/5 mL) has been factored into the unit path and correctly placed so that the wanted unit (mL) correlates with the *wanted quantity* (mL) and the unwanted unit (mg) is canceled from the problem.

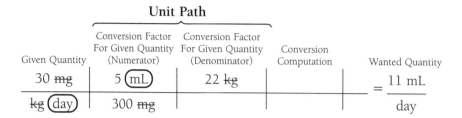

Given Quantity	Conversion Factor For Given Quantity (Numerator)	Conversion Factor For Given Quantity (Denominator)	Conversion Computation	Wanted Quantity
30 m̶g̶	5 (mL)	22 k̶g̶		= 11 mL
k̶g̶ (day)	300 m̶g̶			day

• • • • • THINKING THROUGH THE PROBLEM

The child's weight (22 kg) has been factored into the unit path and set up correctly to allow the unwanted unit (kg) to be canceled from the problem.

Unit Path

Given Quantity	Conversion Factor For Given Quantity (Numerator)	Conversion Factor For Given Quantity (Denominator)	Conversion Computation	Wanted Quantity
30 m̶g̶	5 (mL)	22 k̶g̶	3 × 5 × 22	330	= 11 mL
k̶g̶ (day)	300 m̶g̶		30	30	day

• • • • • THINKING THROUGH THE PROBLEM

All the unwanted units have been canceled from the unit path and the wanted units are correctly placed to correlate with the two-factor–wanted quantity (mL/day). Multiply numerators, multiply denominators, and divide the product of the numerators by the product of the denominators to provide the numerical answer to the problem. The wanted quantity is 11 mL/day.

Using dimensional analysis, calculate how many milliliters per dose the child should receive.

Given quantity = 11 mL/day

Wanted quantity = mL/dose

$$\frac{11 \text{ mL}}{\text{day}} \bigg| \underline{\hspace{7cm}} = \frac{\text{mL}}{\text{dose}}$$

• • • • • THINKING THROUGH THE PROBLEM

The child is to receive 11 mL/day in four divided doses; therefore, the *conversion factor* involves how many doses are in a day (4 divided doses = day).

$$\frac{11 \text{ (mL)}}{\text{day}} \bigg| \frac{\text{day}}{4 \text{ (doses)}} \bigg| \frac{11}{4} = 2.75 \text{ or } \frac{2.8 \text{ mL}}{\text{dose}}$$

The wanted quantity is 2.8 mL/dose and the child will receive this orally (PO) four times a day (qid).

The problem could have been set up to find the wanted quantity of milliliters per dose.

Given quantity = 30 mg/kg/day

Wanted quantity = mL/dose

Dose on hand = 300 mg/5 mL

Weight = 22 kg

Sequential method:

$$\frac{30 \text{ mg}}{\text{kg/day}} \bigg| \frac{5 \text{ (mL)}}{300 \text{ mg}} \bigg| \frac{22 \text{ kg}}{4 \text{ (doses)}} \bigg| \frac{\text{day}}{} \bigg| \frac{3 \times 5 \times 22}{30 \times 4} \frac{330}{120} = 2.75 \text{ or } \frac{2.8 \text{ mL}}{\text{dose}}$$

The wanted quantity is 2.8 mL/dose, and the child will receive this orally (PO) four times a day (qid).

Problem Example #2

As a prudent nurse, you are concerned that the child may be receiving an unsafe dosage of Tagamet, therefore you want to identify how many milligrams per kilogram per day (mg/kg/day) the child weighing 22 kg is receiving. The dosage of medication being given four times a day is 2.8

mL/dose. The dosage on hand is 300 mg/5 mL. How many milligrams per kilogram per day is the child receiving?

Given quantity   = 2.8 mL/dose

Wanted quantity = mg/kg/dose

Dose on hand   = 300 mg/5 mL

Child's weight   = 22 kg

Sequential method:

$$\frac{2.8 \text{ mL}}{\text{dose}} \quad\bigg| \qquad\qquad\qquad = \frac{\text{mg}}{\text{kg/day}}$$

• • • • • THINKING THROUGH THE PROBLEM

The *two-factor–given quantity* (2.8 mL/dose) has been correctly factored into the unit path with a *numerator* (2.8 mL) and a *denominator* (dose). The *three-factor–wanted quantity* (mg/kg/day) also has been correctly factored into the unit path with a *numerator* (mg) and two *denominators* (kg/day).

$$\frac{2.8 \text{ mL}}{\text{dose}} \bigg| \frac{300}{5 \text{ mL}} \bigg| \frac{\text{mg} \bigg| 4 \text{ doses}}{\text{day} \bigg| 22 \text{ kg}} = \frac{\text{mg}}{\text{kg/day}}$$

• • • • • THINKING THROUGH THE PROBLEM

The *conversion factors* have been added to the unit path and all unwanted units have been canceled from the problem. The wanted unit (mg) is correctly placed in the numerator portion of the problem to correlate with the *wanted quantity* (mg) also in the numerator portion of the three-factor–wanted quantity. The wanted units (kg and day) are in the denominator portion of the problem to correlate with the wanted quantity (kg and day) in the denominator portion of the three-factor–wanted quantity.

$$\frac{2.8 \text{ mL} \mid 300 \text{ (mg)} \mid 4 \text{ doses} \mid}{\text{dose} \mid 5 \text{ mL} \mid \text{(day)} \mid 22 \text{ (kg)}} \quad \frac{2.8 \times 300 \times 4 \mid 3360}{5 \times 22 \mid 110} = \frac{30.54 \text{ or } 30.5 \text{ mg}}{\text{kg/day}}$$

The three-factor–wanted quantity is 30.5 mg/kg/day.

• • • • • • **THINKING THROUGH THE PROBLEM**

The nursing drug reference identifies that 20 to 40 mg/kg per day in four divided doses is a safe dosage of Tagamet for children. Therefore, the nurse is assured that the child is receiving a correct dosage. Dimensional analysis assists the learner to critically think through any type of medication problem.

Problem Example #3

The physician orders dobutamine 5 mcg/kg/min IV for cardiac failure. The pharmacy sends an IV bag labeled: dobutamine 250 mg/50 mL D5W/0.45% NS. The patient weighs 165 lb. Calculate the milliliters per hour at which to set the IV pump.

Given quantity = 5 mcg/kg/min

Wanted quantity = mL/hr

Dose on hand = 250 mg/50 mL

Weight = 165 lb

• • • • • • **THINKING THROUGH THE PROBLEM**

Identify the *three-factor–given quantity* (the physician's order) containing three parts, including the *numerator* (5 mg) and *two denominators* (kg/min). Establish the unit path from the three-factor–given quantity to the two-factor–wanted quantity (mL/hr).

Random method:

$$\frac{5 \text{ mcg}}{\text{kg/min}} \bigg| = \frac{\text{mL}}{\text{hr}}$$

●●●●● **THINKING THROUGH THE PROBLEM**

The three-factor–given quantity has been set up correctly with a *numerator* (5 mg) and *two denominators* (kg/min) leading across the unit path to a two-factor–wanted quantity with a *numerator* (mL) and a *denominator* (hr). By using the random method of dimensional analysis the *conversion factors* are factored into the unit path to cancel out unwanted units.

$$\frac{5 \text{ mcg}}{\text{kg/}\cancel{\text{min}}} \bigg| \frac{60 \cancel{\text{min}}}{1 \text{ hr}} = \frac{\text{mL}}{\text{hr}}$$

●●●●● **THINKING THROUGH THE PROBLEM**

The unwanted unit (min) has been canceled from the unit path by factoring the *conversion factor* (1 hr = 60 min), and the wanted unit correctly corresponds with the *wanted quantity denominator* (hr).

$$\frac{5 \text{ mcg}}{\text{kg/}\cancel{\text{min}}} \bigg| \frac{60 \cancel{\text{min}}}{1 \text{ (hr)}} \bigg| \frac{50 \text{ (mL)}}{250 \text{ mg}} = \frac{\text{mL}}{\text{hr}}$$

●●●●● **THINKING THROUGH THE PROBLEM**

The *dose on hand* (250 mg/50 mL) has been factored into the unit path and placed so that the *wanted unit* (mL) correctly corresponds with the wanted quantity numerator (mL).

$$\frac{5 \; \cancel{mcg}}{kg/\cancel{min}} \bigg| \frac{60 \; \cancel{min}}{1 \; \cancelcircle{hr}} \bigg| \frac{50 \; \cancelcircle{mL}}{250 \; \cancel{mg}} \bigg| \frac{1 \; \cancel{mg}}{1000 \; \cancel{mcg}} = \frac{mL}{hr}$$

• • • • • **THINKING THROUGH THE PROBLEM**

The *conversion factor* (1 mg = 1000 mcg) has been factored into the unit path to cancel the unwanted units (mg and mcg).

$$\frac{5 \; \cancel{mcg}}{\cancel{kg/min}} \bigg| \frac{60 \; \cancel{min}}{1 \; \cancelcircle{hr}} \bigg| \frac{50 \; \cancelcircle{mL}}{250 \; \cancel{mg}} \bigg| \frac{1 \; \cancel{mg}}{1000 \; \cancel{mcg}} \bigg| \frac{1 \; \cancel{kg}}{2.2 \; \cancel{lb}} \bigg| 165 \; \cancel{lb} = \frac{mL}{hr}$$

• • • • • **THINKING THROUGH THE PROBLEM**

The final *conversion factors* (1 kg = 2.2 lb) and the *weight* of the patient have been factored into the unit path to cancel the remaining unwanted units (kg and lb). All the unwanted units have been canceled from the unit path and the wanted units (mL and hr) remain in the unit path in the correct positions to correlate with the *two-factor–wanted quantity* (mL/hr). Multiply the numerators, multiply the denominators, and divide the product of the numerators by the product of the denominators to provide the numerical value for the two-factor–wanted quantity.

$$\frac{5 \; \cancel{mcg}}{\cancel{kg/min}} \bigg| \frac{\cancel{60 \; min}}{\cancel{1} \; \cancelcircle{hr}} \bigg| \frac{50 \; \cancelcircle{mL}}{\cancel{250} \; \cancel{mg}} \bigg| \frac{1 \; \cancel{mg}}{\cancel{1000} \; \cancel{mcg}} \bigg| \frac{1 \; \cancel{kg}}{2.2 \; \cancel{lb}} \bigg| 165 \; \cancel{lb} = \frac{mL}{hr}$$

$$\frac{5 \times 6 \times 5 \times 1 \times 165}{25 \times 100 \times 2.2} \bigg| \frac{24750}{5500} = \frac{4.5 \; mL}{hr}$$

• • • • • • **THINKING THROUGH THE PROBLEM**

The wanted quantity is 4.5 mL/hr and is the answer to the problem. Intravenous pumps used in critical care can be set to deliver amounts including decimal points so it is not necessary to round up the answer.

Problem Example #4

The nurse has been monitoring the hemodynamic readings of a patient weighing 165 lb receiving dobutamine, 250 mg in 50 mL of D5W/0.45% NS, and has received additional orders from the physician to *titrate* for effectiveness. The IV pump is now set at 9 mL/hr, and the physician wants to know how many micrograms per kilogram per minute the patient is now receiving.

Given quantity   = 9 mL/hr

Wanted quantity = mcg/kg/min

Dose on hand   = 250 mg/50 mL

Weight   = 165 lb

$$\frac{9 \text{ mL}}{\text{hr}} \bigg| \qquad\qquad\qquad\qquad\qquad = \frac{\text{mcg}}{\text{kg/min}}$$

• • • • • • **THINKING THROUGH THE PROBLEM**

The *two-factor–given quantity* is identified as the information that the nurse obtained from the IV pump, and the *three-factor–wanted quantity* is the information that the physician has requested.

Sequential method:

$$\frac{9 \text{ mL}}{\text{hr}} \bigg| \frac{250 \text{ mg}}{50 \text{ mL}} \qquad\qquad = \frac{\text{mcg}}{\text{kg/min}}$$

•••••• THINKING THROUGH THE PROBLEM

The *dose on hand* (the IV fluid that is presently infusing) has been factored into the unit path to cancel the unwanted unit (mL) from the problem.

$$\frac{9 \text{ mL}}{\text{hr}} \left| \frac{250 \text{ mg}}{50 \text{ mL}} \right| \frac{1000 \text{ mcg}}{1 \text{ mg}} = \frac{\text{mcg}}{\text{kg/min}}$$

•••••• THINKING THROUGH THE PROBLEM

The *conversion factor* (1 mg = 1000 mcg) has been factored into the unit path to cancel the unwanted unit (mg) from the problem. The wanted unit (mcg) remains in the unit path and correctly corresponds with the wanted quantity in the *numerator* portion of the problem.

$$\frac{9 \text{ mL}}{\text{hr}} \left| \frac{250 \text{ mg}}{50 \text{ mL}} \right| \frac{1000 \text{ mcg}}{1 \text{ mg}} \left| \frac{1 \text{ hr}}{60 \text{ min}} \right| = \frac{\text{mcg}}{\text{kg/min}}$$

•••••• THINKING THROUGH THE PROBLEM

The *conversion factor* (1 hr = 60 min) has been factored into the unit path to cancel the unwanted unit (hr) from the problem. The wanted unit (min) remains in the unit path correctly placed in the *denominator* portion of the problem.

$$\frac{9 \text{ mL}}{\text{hr}} \left| \frac{250 \text{ mg}}{50 \text{ mL}} \right| \frac{1000 \text{ mcg}}{1 \text{ mg}} \left| \frac{1 \text{ hr}}{60 \text{ min}} \right| \frac{2.2 \text{ lb}}{1 \text{ kg}} \left| 165 \text{ lb} \right| = \frac{\text{mcg}}{\text{kg/min}}$$

• • • • • **THINKING THROUGH THE PROBLEM**

> The *conversion factor* (1 kg = 2.2 lb) has been factored into the unit path to correspond with the *wanted quantity denominator* (kg). The *weight* of the patient also is factored into the unit path to cancel the unwanted unit (lb) from the problem. After all unwanted units have been canceled from the problem and the wanted units correctly identified, multiply the numerators, multiply the denominators, and divide the product of the numerators by the product of the denominators to provide the numerical value for the *wanted quantity*.

$$\frac{9 \text{ mL}}{\text{hr}} \bigg| \frac{250 \text{ mg}}{50 \text{ mL}} \bigg| \frac{1000 \text{ mcg}}{1 \text{ mg}} \bigg| \frac{1 \text{ hr}}{60 \text{ min}} \bigg| \frac{2.2 \text{ lb}}{1 \text{ kg}} \bigg| \frac{}{165 \text{ lb}} = \frac{\text{mcg}}{\text{kg/min}}$$

$$\frac{9 \times 25 \times 100 \times 2.2}{5 \times 6 \times 1 \times 165} \bigg| \frac{49500}{4950} = \frac{10 \text{ mcg}}{\text{kg/min}}$$

The nurse can inform the physician that the patient is now receiving 10 mcg/kg/min infusing at 9 mL/hr.

Dimensional analysis is a problem-solving method that uses critical thinking. When implementing the *sequential method* or the *random method* of dimensional analysis, the medication problem can be set up in a number of different ways, with a focus on the correct placement of *conversion factors* to allow unwanted units to be canceled from the unit path.

Dimensional analysis is a problem-solving method that nurses can use to calculate a variety of medication problems in the hospital, outpatient, or the home-care environment. The medication problems may involve one-factor–, two-factor–, or three-factor–given quantity medication orders, resulting in one-factor–, two-factor–, or three-factor–wanted quantity answers.

With advanced nursing and home-care nursing resulting in increased autonomy, it is more important than ever that nurses be able to accurately calculate medication problems. Dimensional analysis provides the opportunity to use one problem-solving method for any type of medication problem, thereby increasing consistency and decreasing confusion when calculating medication problems.

Practice Problems Involving Dosage, Weight, and Time

1. Order: furosemide, 2 mg/kg per day PO in two divided doses, for congestive heart failure.
   Supply: furosemide 40 mg/5 mL
   Child's weight: 20 kg
   How many milliliters per dose will you give?

Figure 6-1. Furosemide. (Courtesy of Roxane Laboratories)

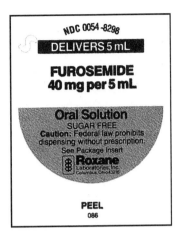

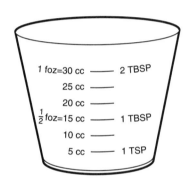

2. Order: Ancef, 40 mg/kg/day in divided doses every 8 hours, for infection.
   Supply: Ancef 1 g
   Child's weight: 30 lb
   Nursing drug reference: Reconstitute with 10 mL of sterile water for injection.
   How many milliliters per dose will you draw from the vial after reconstitution?

Figure 6-2. Ancef®/Cefazolin sodium. (Courtesy of Smith-Kline Beecham Pharmaceuticals)

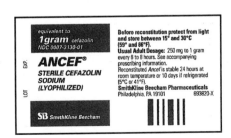

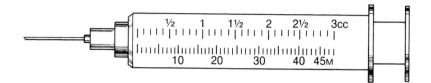

3. Order: Dilantin, 6 mg/kg/day in divided doses every 12 hours, for seizures.
   Supply: Dilantin 125 mg/5 mL
   Child's weight: 45 lb
   How many milliliters per dose will you give?

4. Order: prednisone, 1.5 mg/kg/day in four divided doses, for inflammation.
   Supply: prednisone 6.7 mg/5 mL
   Child's weight: 20 kg
   How many milliliters per dose will you give?

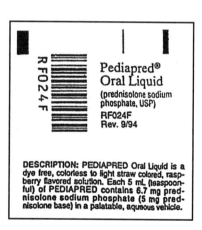

Figure 6-3. Pediapred®/prednisolone sodium phosphate package insert. (Courtesy of Fisons Pharmaceuticals)

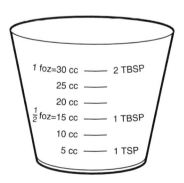

5. Order: Cleocin, 10 mg/kg/day IV in divided doses every 8 hours, for infection.
   Supply: Cleocin 300 mg/2 mL
   Child's weight: 50 lb
   How many milliliters per dose will you give?

Figure 6-4. Cleocin®/clindamycin phosphate package insert. (Courtesy of the Upjohn Company)

Upjohn

Cleocin Phosphate®
brand of clindamycin phosphate sterile solution and clindamycin phosphate IV solution
(clindamycin phosphate injection, USP and clindamycin phosphate injection in 5% dextrose)
Sterile Solution is for Intramuscular and Intravenous Use
CLEOCIN PHOSPHATE in the ADD-Vantage™ Vial is For Intravenous Use Only

DESCRIPTION
   CLEOCIN PHOSPHATE Sterile Solution in vials contains clindamycin phosphate, a water soluble ester of clindamycin and phosphoric acid. Each mL contains the equivalent of 150 mg clindamycin, 0.5 mg disodium edetate and 9.45 mg benzyl alcohol added as preservative in each mL. Clindamycin is a semisynthetic antibiotic produced by a 7(S)-chloro-substitution of the 7(R)-hydroxyl group of the parent compound lincomycin.

6. Order: dopamine, 5 mcg/kg/min IV, to increase blood pressure.
   Supply: Dopamine 400-mg vial
   Supply: 250 cc D$_5$W
   Patient's weight: 200 lb
   How many milliliters will you draw from the vial?
   Calculate milliliters per hour to set the IV pump.

Figure 6-5. Dopamine HCl. (Courtesy of Astra Pharmaceutical Products)

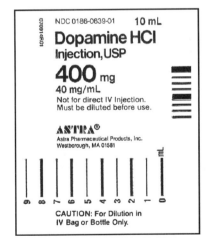

NDC 0186-0639-01   10 mL
Dopamine HCl
Injection, USP
400 mg
40 mg/mL
Not for direct IV Injection.
Must be diluted before use.

ASTRA®
Astra Pharmaceutical Products, Inc.
Westborough, MA 01581

CAUTION: For Dilution in
IV Bag or Bottle Only.

Dopamine Hydrochloride Injection, USP

DOSAGE AND ADMINISTRATION
WARNING: This is a potent drug. It must be diluted before administration to patient.

Suggested Dilution
Transfer contents of one or more additive syringes of dopamine hydrochloride by aseptic technique to either a 250 mL, or 500 mL container of one of the following sterile intravenous solutions:

1. Sodium Chloride Injection, USP
2. Dextrose 5% Injection, USP
3. Dextrose (5%) and Sodium Chloride (0.9%) Injection, USP
4. Dextrose (5%) and Sodium Chloride (0.45%) Injection, USP
5. Dextrose (5%) in Lactated Ringer's Injection
6. Sodium Lactate (1/6 Molar) Injection, USP
7. Lactated Ringer's Injection, USP

Dopamine HCl has been found to be stable for a minimum of 24 hours after dilution in the sterile intravenous solutions listed above. However, as with all intravenous admixtures, dilution should be made just prior to administration.

Do NOT add dopamine HCl to 5% Sodium Bicarbonate or other alkaline intravenous solution, since the drug is inactivated in alkaline solution.

Rate of Administration
Dopamine HCl, after dilution, is administered intravenously through a suitable intravenous catheter or needle. An IV drip chamber or other suitable metering device is essential for controlling the rate of flow in drops/minute. Each patient must be individually titrated to the desired hemodynamic and/or renal response with dopamine HCl. In titrating to the desired increase in systolic blood pressure, the optimum dosage rate for renal response may be exceeded, thus necessitating a reduction in rate after the hemodynamic condition is stabilized.

Administration at rates greater than 50 mcg/kg/minute have safely been used in advanced circulatory decompensation states. If unnecessary fluid expansion is of concern, adjustment of drug concentration may be preferred over increasing the flow rate of a less concentrated dilution.

Suggested Regimen
1. When appropriate, increase blood volume with whole blood or plasma until central venous pressure is 10 to 15 cm H_2O or pulmonary wedge pressure is 14 to 18 mm Hg.
2. Begin administration of diluted solution at doses of 2–5 mcg/kg/minute dopamine HCl in patients who are likely to respond to modest increments of heart force and renal perfusion.
   In more seriously ill patients, begin administration of diluted solution at doses of 5 mcg/kg/minute dopamine HCl and increase gradually using 5–10 mcg/kg/minute increments up to 20–50 mcg/kg/minute as needed. If doses of dopamine HCl in excess of 50 mcg/kg/minute are required, it is suggested that urine output be checked frequently. Should urine flow begin to decrease in the absence of hypotension, reduction of dopamine HCl dosage should be considered. Multiclinic trials have shown that more than 50% of the patients were satisfactorily maintained on doses of dopamine HCl of less than 20 mcg/kg/minute. In patients who do not respond to these doses with adequate arterial pressures or urine flow, additional increments of dopamine HCl may be employed in an effort to produce an appropriate arterial pressure and central perfusion.
3. Treatment of all patients requires constant evaluation of therapy in terms of the blood volume, augmentation of myocardial contractility, and distribution of peripheral perfusion. Dosage of dopamine HCl should be adjusted according to the patient's response, with particular attention to diminution of established urine flow rate, increasing tachycardia or development of new dysrhythmias as indices for decreasing or temporarily suspending the dosage.
4. As with all potent administered drugs, care should be taken to control the rate of administration to avoid inadvertent administration of a bolus of drug.

Parenteral drug products should be inspected visually for particulate matter and discoloration prior to administration, whenever solution and container permit.

HOW SUPPLIED
Dopamine HCl 200 mg is supplied in the following form:
Additive Syringe   5 mL (40 mg/mL)   NDC 0186-0638-01

Dopamine HCl 400 mg is supplied in the following forms:
Additive Syringe   5 mL (80 mg/mL)   NDC 0186-0641-01
                   10 mL (40 mg/mL)   NDC 0186-0639-01

Dopamine HCl 800 mg is supplied in the following form:
Additive Syringe   5 mL (160 mg/mL)   NDC 0186-0642-01

Packages are color coded according to the total dosage content; 200 mg coded blue/white, 400 mg coded green/white and 800 mg coded yellow/white.

Store at controlled room temperature 15°–30°C (59°–86°F). Protect from light.

Avoid contact with alkalies (including sodium bicarbonate), oxidizing agents, or iron salts.

NOTE: Do not use the Injection if it is darker than slightly yellow or discolored in any way.

ASTRA® | Astra Pharmaceutical Products, Inc.
             Westborough, MA 01581

021861R07   3/92 (7)

Figure 6-6. Dopamine package insert. (Courtesy of Astra Pharmaceutical Products)

7. Information obtained by the nurse: Nipride, 50 mg/250 mL D5W is infusing at 22 mL/hr.
   Patient's weight: 160 lb
   How many micrograms per kilogram per minute is the patient receiving?

8. Order: Inocor, 5 mcg/kg/min IV for congestive heart failure.
   Supply: Inocor 100 mg/100 mL of 0.9% NS
   Patient's weight: 180 lb
   Calculate milliliters per hour to set the IV pump.

9. Information obtained by the nurse: Nipride, 50 mg/250 mL D5W, is infusing at 46 mL/hr.
   Patient's weight: 160 lb
   How many micrograms per kilogram per minute is the patient receiving?

10. Order: bretylium, 5 mg/kg in 50 mL D_5W i.v. over 30 minutes, for arrhythmia.
    Supply: bretylium 500-mg vial
    Patient's weight: 240 lb
    How many milliliters will you draw from the vial?
    Calculate milliliters per hour to set the IV pump.

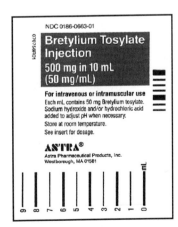

Figure 6-7. Bretylium tosylate. (Courtesy of Astra Pharmaceutical Products)

Bretylium Tosylate Injection
For Intramuscular or Intravenous Use.

Suggested Bretylium Tosylate Admixture Dilutions and Administration Rates
for Continuous Infusion Maintenance Therapy Arranged in Descending Order of Concentration

	PREPARATION			ADMINISTRATION		
Amount of Bretylium Tosylate	Volume of IV Fluid*	Final Volume	Final conc. (mg/mL)	Dose mg/min	Microdrops per min	mL/hour
FOR FLUID RESTRICTED PATIENTS:						
500 mg (10 mL)	50 mL	60 mL	8.3	1.0	7	7
				1.5	11	11
				2.0	14	14
2 g (40 mL)	500 mL	540 mL	3.7	1.0	16	16
1 g (20 mL)	250 mL	270 mL	3.7	1.5	24	24
				2.0	32	32
1 g (20 mL)	500 mL	520 mL	1.9	1.0	32	32
500 mg (10 mL)	250 mL	260 mL	1.9	1.5	47	47
				2.0	63	63

*IV fluid may be either Dextrose Injection, USP or Sodium Chloride Injection, USP. This table does not consider the overfill volume present in the IV fluids.

Figure 6-8. Bretylium tosylate package insert. (Courtesy of Astra Pharmaceutical Products)

This chapter has assisted the learner to calculate three-factor medication problems involving the *dosage* of medication, the *weight* of the patient, and the amount of *time* over which medications or intravenous fluids can be safely administered. Using the sequential method or the random method of dimensional analysis, demonstrate your ability to calculate medication problems accurately by completing the following practice problems.

Practice Problems

1. Order: amrinone, 8 mcg/kg/min IV, for congestive heart failure.
   Supply: amrinone 100 mg/100 mL of 0.9% NS
   Patient's weight: 198 lb
   Calculate milliliters per hour to set the IV pump.

2. Order: Tagamet, 40 mg/kg/day PO in four divided doses, for gastrointestinal ulcers.
   Supply: Tagamet 300 mg/5 mL
   Child's weight: 80 lb
   How many milliliters per dose will you give?

3. Information obtained by the nurse: dopamine, 200 mg in 500 mL D5W, is infusing at 45 mL/hr for a patient weighing 60 kg.
   How many micrograms per kilogram per minute is the patient receiving?

4. Order: dopamine, 2 mcg/kg/min IV, for decreased cardiac output.
   Supply: dopamine 400 mg/500 mL
   Patient's weight: 176 lb
   Calculate milliliters per hour to set the IV pump.

5. Order: Neupogen, 5 mcg/kg/day sq for 2 weeks, for neutropenia.
   Supply: Neupogen 300 mcg/mL
   Patient's weight: 130 lb
   How many micrograms per day will you give?

6. Order: aminophylline, 0.5 mg/kg/hr IV loading dose, for bronchodilation.
   Supply: aminophylline 250 mg/250 mL D5W
   Patient's weight: 132 lb
   Calculate milliliters per hour to set the IV pump.

7. Order: furosemide, 2 mg/kg per day PO, for congestive heart failure.
   Supply: furosemide 10 mg/mL
   Child's weight: 40 kg
   How many milliliters per day will you give?

8. Information obtained by the nurse: Nipride, 200 mg in 1000 mL D5W, is infusing at 15 mL/hr for a patient weighing 100 kg.
   How many micrograms per kilogram per minute is the patient receiving?

9. Information obtained by the nurse: A child weighing 65 lb is receiving 10 mL of Taga-met PO qid from a stock bottle labeled: Tagamet, 300 mg/5 mL.
   How many milligrams per kilogram per day is the child receiving?

10. Information obtained by the nurse: aminophylline, 250 mg/250 mL 0.9% NS, is infus-ing at 25 mL/hr for a patient weighing 50 kg.
    How many milligrams per kilogram per hour is the patient receiving?

7

Practicing Problems With Dimensional Analysis

This chapter will allow the learner to practice calculating one-factor, two-factor, and three-factor medication problems using dimensional analysis. The goal of this chapter is to demonstrate that the learner has a clear understanding of dimensional analysis as a problem-solving method and is capable of accurately solving a variety of medication problems.

One-Factor Practice Problems

1. Order: Tigan, 200 mg qid IM, for nausea and vomiting.
   How many milliliters will you give?

Figure 7-1. Tigan®/trimethobenzamide HCl. (Courtesy of SmithKline Beecham Pharmaceuticals)

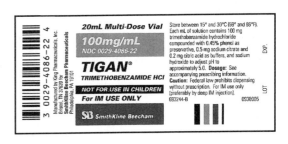

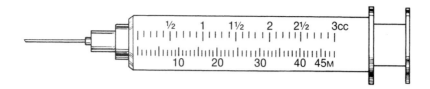

2. Order: morphine, 30 mg PO every 4 hours, for pain.
   How many tablets will you give?

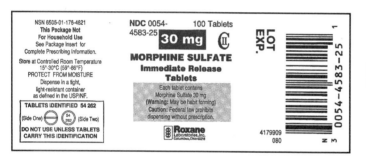

Figure 7-2. Morphine sulfate. (Courtesy of Roxane Laboratories)

3. Order: prednisone, 7.5 mg PO bid, for inflammation.
   How many tablets will you give?

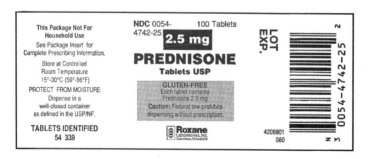

Figure 7-3. Prednisone. (Courtesy of Roxane Laboratories)

4. Order: acetaminophen, 160 mg PO every 4 hours, for fever.
   How many teaspoons will you give?

Figure 7-4. Acetaminophen. (Courtesy of Roxane Laboratories)

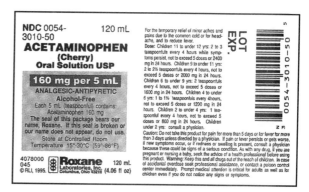

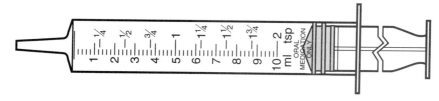

5. Order: Xanax, 0.5 mg PO tid, for anxiety.
   How many tablets will you give?

Figure 7-5. Xanax®/alprazolam. (Courtesy of the Upjohn Company)

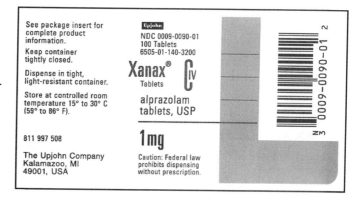

6. Order: Adalat, 60 mg PO, daily for hypertension.
   How many tablets will you give?

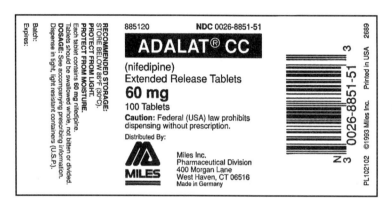

Figure 7-6. Adalat®/nifedipine. (Courtesy of Miles Inc.)

7. Order: Halcion, 0.25 mg PO at hs, for insomnia.
   How many tablets will you give?

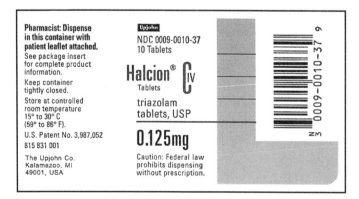

Figure 7-7. Halcion®/triazolam. (Courtesy of the Upjohn Company)

8. Order: furosemide, 80 mg PO daily, for congestive heart failure.
   How many tablets will you give?

Figure 7-8. Furosemide. (Courtesy of Roxane Laboratories)

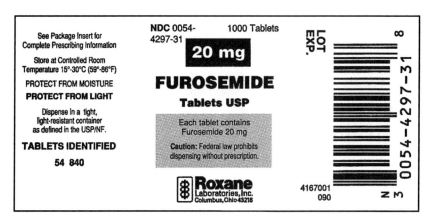

9. Order: morphine sulfate, 10 mg IM prn, for pain.
   How many milliliters will you give?

Figure 7-9. Morphine sulfate. (Courtesy of Astra Pharmaceutical Products)

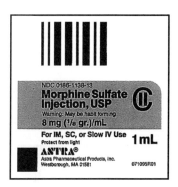

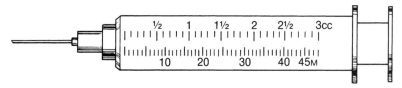

10. Order: naloxone HCl, 100 mcg IVP prn, for respiratory depression.
   How many milliliters will you give?

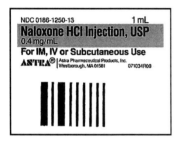

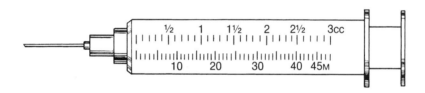

Figure 7-10. Naloxone HCl. (Courtesy of Astra Pharmaceutical Products)

11. Order: Solu-Medrol, 80 mg IVP every 4 hours, for inflammation.
   How many milliliters will you give?

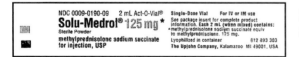

Figure 7-11. Solu-Medrol®/methylprednisolone. (Courtesy of the Upjohn Company)

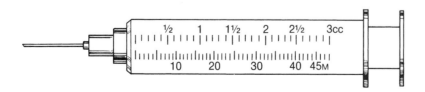

12. Order: lactulose, 20 g PO daily, for constipation.
    How many milliliters will you give?

Figure 7-12. Lactulose. (Courtesy of Roxane Laboratories)

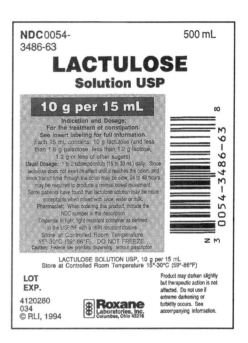

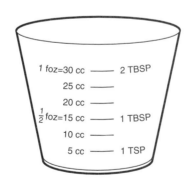

13. Order: Compazine, 5 mg IM tid, for nausea and vomiting.
    How many milliliters will you give?

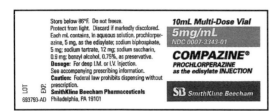

Figure 7-13. Compazine®/prochlorperazine. (Courtesy of SmithKline Beecham Pharmaceuticals)

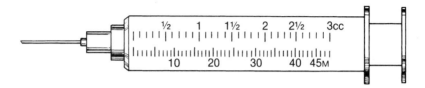

14. Order: Augmentin, 250 mg PO every 8 hours, for infection. How many milliliters will you give?

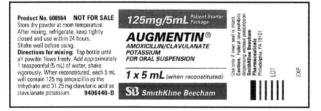

Figure 7-14. Augmentin®/amoxicillin. (Courtesy of SmithKline Beecham Pharmaceuticals)

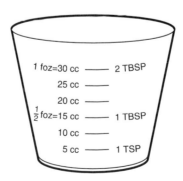

15. Order: Tigan, 200 mg PO tid, for nausea and vomiting.
    How many capsules will you give?

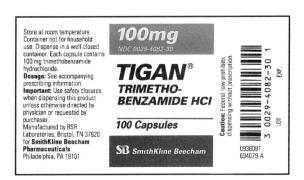

Figure 7-15. Tigan®/trimethobenzamide HCl. (Courtesy of SmithKline Beecham Pharmaceuticals)

16. Order: prednisone, 10 mg PO bid, for adrenal insufficiency.
    How many tablets will you give?

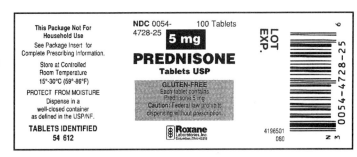

Figure 7-16. Prednisone. (Courtesy of Roxane Laboratories)

17. Order: hydromorphone, 3 mg IM every 4 hours, for pain.
    How many milliliters will you give?

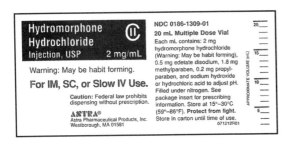

Figure 7-17. Hydromorphone hydrochloride. (Courtesy of Astra Pharmaceutical Products)

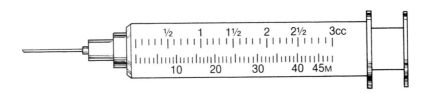

18. Order: acetaminophen, 400 mg PO every 4 hours prn, for fever.
How many milliliters will you give?

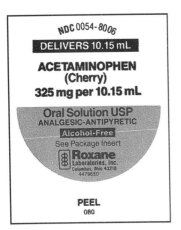

Figure 7-18. Acetaminophen. (Courtesy of Roxane Laboratories)

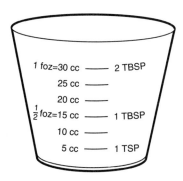

19. Order: magnesium sulfate, 1000 mg IM times four doses, for hypomagnesemia.
    How many milliliters will you give?

Figure 7-19. Magnesium sulfate. (Courtesy of Astra Pharmaceutical Products)

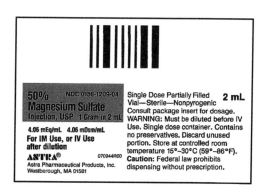

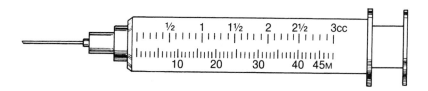

20. Order: Compazine, 10 mg PO qid prn, for nausea and vomiting.
    How many teaspoons will you give?

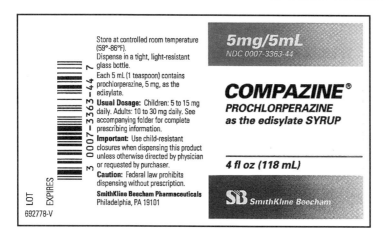

Figure 7-20. Compazine®/prochlorperazine. (Courtesy of Smith-Kline Beecham Pharmaceuticals)

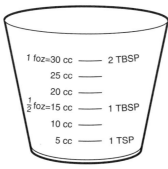

Two-Factor Practice Problems

• •

1. Order: digoxin elixir, 25 mcg/kg, for congestive heart failure.
   Child's weight: 25 lb
   How many milliliters will you give?

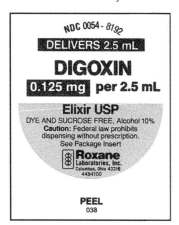

Figure 7-21. Digoxin. (Courtesy of Roxane Laboratories)

2. Order: atropine sulfate, 0.02 mg/kg IV every 4 hours, for bradycardia.
   Child's weight: 35 lb
   How many milliliters will you give?

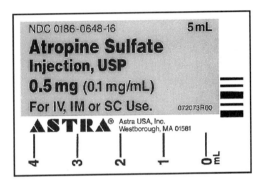

Figure 7-22. Atropine sulfate. (Courtesy of Astra Pharmaceutical Products)

3. Order: lidocaine, 2 mg/min IV, for arrhythmia.
   Supply: lidocaine 2 g/500 mL D5W
   Calculate milliliters per hour to set the IV pump.

4. Order: Mezlin, 1.5 g IV every 4 hours, for infection.
   Nursing drug reference: Reconstitute each 1 g with 10 mL of normal saline.
   How many milliliters will you draw from the vial after reconstitution?

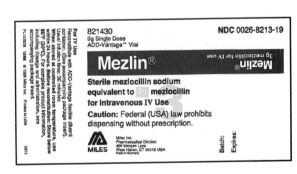

Figure 7-23. Mezlin®/mezlocillin sodium. (Courtesy of Miles)

5. Order: gentamicin, 1 mg/kg IV every 8 hours, for infection.
   Supply: gentamicin 40 mg/mL
   Child's weight: 94 lb
   How many milliliters will you draw from the vial?

6. Order: morphine, 15 mg/hr IV, for intractable pain.
   Supply: morphine 300 mg/500 mL NS
   Calculate milliliters per hour to set the IV pump.

7. Information obtained by the nurse: Dilaudid, 50 mg in 250 mL NS is infusing at 25 mL/hr.
   How many milligrams per hour is the patient receiving?

8. Order: add 10 mEq KCl to 1000 mL D5W
   Supply: KCl 20 mEq/20 mL
   How many milliliters will you draw from the vial to add to the IV bag?

9. Information obtained by the nurse: nitroglycerin, 50 mg in 500 mL D5W, is infusing at 3 mL/hr.
   How many micrograms per minute is the patient receiving?

10. Information obtained by the nurse: 1000 mL D5W with 10 mEq KCl is infusing at 100 mL/hr.
    How many milliequivalents of KCl is the patient receiving per hour?

11. Order: infuse 1000 mL D5W at 250 mL/hr
    Drop factor: 20 gtt/mL
    Calculate the number of drops per minute.

12. Order: infuse 750 mL NS over 5 hours.
    Drop factor: 10 gtt/mL
    Calculate the number of drops per minute.

13. Order: infuse 500 mL D5W over 8 hours.
    Drop factor: 60 gtt/mL
    Calculate the number of drops per minute.

14. Order: infuse 750 mL D5W
    Drop factor: 15 gtt/mL
    Infusion rate: 18 gtt/min
    Calculate the number of hours to infuse.

15. Order: infuse 250 mL NS
    Drop factor: 15 gtt/mL
    Infusion rate: 50 gtt/min
    Calculate the number of hours to infuse.

16. Order: infuse 1000 mL D5W/0.45% NS.
    Drop factor: 15 gtt/mL
    Infusion rate: 25 gtt/min
    Calculate the number of hours to infuse.

17. Order: Fortaz, 1.25 g IV every 12 hours, for urinary tract infection.
Supply: Fortaz 2-g vial
Nursing drug reference: Dilute each 1 g with 10 mL of sterile water and further dilute in 100 mL 0.9% NS to infuse over 1 hour.
How many milliliters will you draw from the vial after reconstitution?
Calculate the milliliters per hour to set the IV pump.
Calculate the drops per minute with a drop factor of 10 gtt/mL.

18. Order: vancomycin, 275 mg IV every 8 hours, for infection.
Supply: Vancomycin 500-mg vial
Nursing drug reference: Reconstitute each 500-mg vial with 10 mL NS and further dilute with 250 mL NS to infuse over 1 hour.
How many milliliters will you draw from the vial after reconstitution?
Calculate milliliters per hour to set the IV pump.
Calculate the drops per minute with a drop factor of 10 gtt/mL.

19. Order: Mezlin, 450 mg IV every 4 hours, for infection
Supply: Mezlin 4-g vial
Nursing drug reference: Reconstitute each 1 g with 10 mL of sterile water and further dilute in 100 mL NS to infuse over 30 min.
How many milliliters will you draw from the vial after reconstitution?
Calculate milliliters per hour to set the IV pump.
Calculate drops per minute with a drop factor of 10 gtt/mL.

20. Order: gentamicin, 23 mg IV every 8 hours, for infection
Supply: gentamicin 40 mg/mL
Nursing drug reference: Dilute with 100 mL NS and infuse over 1 hour.
How many milliliters will you draw from the vial?
Calculate the milliliters per hour to set the IV pump.
Calculate the drops per minute with a drop factor of 15 gtt/mL.

Three-Factor Practice Problems

1. Order: Tagamet, 40 mg/kg/day PO in four divided doses, for treatment of active ulcer
   Child's weight: 60 kg
   How many milliliters per day will you give?
   How many milliliters per dose will you give?

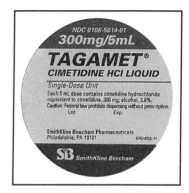

Figure 7-24. Tagamet®/cimetidine HCl. (Courtesy of SmithKline Beecham Pharmaceuticals)

2. Order: furosemide, 4 mg/kg/day IV, for management of hypercalcemia of malignancy.
   Child's weight: 60 lb
   How many milliliters per day will you give?

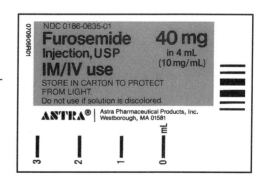

Figure 7-25. Furosemide. (Courtesy of Astra Pharmaceutical Products)

3. Order: Cleocin, 30 mg/kg/day IV in divided doses every 8 hours, for infection
   Child's weight: 50 kg
   How many milliliters per day will you give?
   How many milliliters per dose will you give?

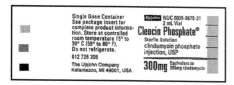

Figure 7-26. Cleocin®/clindamycin phosphate. (Courtesy of the Upjohn Company)

4. Information obtained by the nurse: A child is receiving 0.575 mL/dose of gentamicin IV every 8 hours from a supply of gentamicin 40 mg/mL.
   Child's weight: 45 lb
   How many milligrams per kilogram per day is the child receiving?

5. Information obtained by the nurse: A child is receiving 0.125 mL/dose of diphenhydramine (Benadryl) IV every 8 hours from a supply of Benadryl 50 mg/mL.
   Child's weight: 20 lb
   How many milligrams per kilogram per day is the child receiving?

6. Order: dopamine, 5 mcg/kg/min IV, for decreased cardiac output.
   Supply: dopamine 400-mg vial
   Nursing drug reference: Dilute each 400-mg vial in 250 mL NS
   Patient's weight: 110 lb
   How many milliliters will you draw from the vial?
   Calculate the milliliters per hour to set the IV pump.

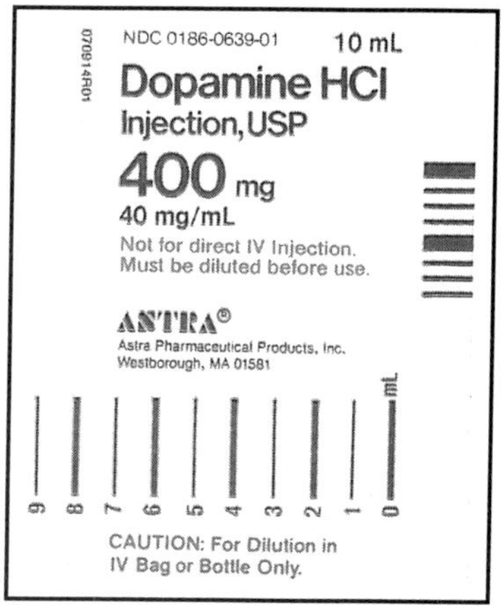

Figure 7-27. Dopamine HCl. (Courtesy of Astra Pharmaceutical Products)

7. Order: Nipride, 0.8 mcg/kg/min IV, for hypertensive crisis.
Supply: Nipride 50 mg/500 mL NS
Patient's weight: 143 lb
Calculate the milliliters per hour to set the IV pump.

8. Information obtained by the nurse: Nipride, 50 mg in 250 mL NS, is infusing at 68 mL/hr.
Patient's weight: 250 lb
How many micrograms per kilogram per minute is the patient receiving?

9. Order: Hydrea, 30 mg/kg/day PO, for ovarian carcinoma
Patient's weight: 157 lb
How many grams per day is the patient receiving?

10. Order: Venoglobulin-S, 0.01 mL/kg/min, for treatment of immunodeficiency syndrome
Patient's weight: 180 lb
Calculate milliliter per hour to set the IV pump.

11. Information obtained by the nurse: dopamine, 400 mg in 250 mL D5W, is infusing at 28 mL/hr
    Patient's weight: 15 kg
    How many micrograms per kilogram per minute is the patient receiving?

12. Order: Inocor, 3 mcg/kg/min IV, for congestive heart failure.
    Supply: Inocor 100 mg/100 mL of 0.9% NS
    Patient's weight: 160 lb
    Calculate milliliters per hour to set the IV pump.

13. Information obtained by the nurse: Nipride, 50 mg in 250 mL NS, is infusing at 68 mL/hr
    Patient's weight: 250 lb
    How many micrograms per kilogram per minute is the patient receiving?

14. Order: Nipride, 1 mcg/kg/min IV, for hypertensive crisis
    Supply: Nipride 50 mg/250 mL NS
    Patient's weight: 160 lb
    Calculate milliliters per hour to set the IV pump

15. Order: dopamine, 2.5 mcg/kg/min IV, for hypotension
    Supply: dopamine 400 mg/500 mL D5W
    Patient's weight: 65 kg
    Calculate milliliters per hour to set the IV pump.

16. Information obtained by the nurse: Isuprel, 2 mg in 500 mL D5W, is infusing at 15 mL/hr.
    Child's weight: 20 kg
    How many micrograms per kilogram per minute is the child receiving?

17. Order: Intropin, 5 mcg/kg/min IV, for treatment of oliguria following shock
    Supply: Intropin 400 mg/500 mL NS
    Patient's weight: 70 kg
    Calculate milliliters per minute.

18. Order: vancomycin, 40 mg/kg/day IV, for infection
    Supply: vancomycin 500-mg vial
    Nursing drug reference: Reconstitute each 500-mg vial with 10 mL sterile water and further dilute in 100 mL of 0.9% NS to infuse over 60 minutes.
    Child's weight: 20 lb
    How many milligrams per day is the child receiving?
    How many milligrams per dose is the child receiving?
    How many milliliters will you draw from the vial after reconstitution?
    Calculate milliliters per hour to set the IV pump.

19. Order: gentamicin, 2 mg/kg/dose IV every 8 hours, for infection
    Supply: gentamicin 40-mg/mL vial
    Nursing drug reference: Further dilute in 50 mL NS and infuse over 30 minutes.
    Child's weight: 40 kg
    How many milligrams per dose is the child receiving?
    How many milliliters will you draw from the vial?
    Calculate milliliters per hour to set the IV pump.

20. Order: Ancef, 25 mg/kg/day IV every 8 hours, for infection
    Supply: Ancef 500-mg vial
    Nursing drug reference: Reconstitute each 500-mg vial with 10 mL of sterile water and further dilute in 50 mL NS to infuse over 30 minutes.
    Child's weight: 25 kg
    How many milligrams per day is the child receiving?
    How many milligrams per dose is the child receiving?
    How many milliliters will you draw from the vial after reconstitution?
    Calculate milliliters per hour to set the IV pump.

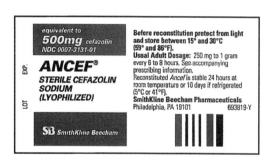

Figure 7-28. Ancef®/cefazolin sodium. (Courtesy of SmithKline Beecham Pharmaceuticals)

This chapter has provided the learner with the opportunity for extensive practice with a variety of medication problems using dimensional analysis as a problem-solving method. It has also provided learners the opportunity to review one-factor, two-factor, and three-factor medication problems to evaluate their comprehension. A review of corresponding chapters and problem examples is provided in the answer section of the chapter to assist the learner in identification of errors with the setup of the problems and to ensure mastery of the concept of dimensional analysis.

8

Comprehensive Post-Test

This chapter includes 20 comprehensive medication calculation problems to permit a self-evaluation of your ability to calculate medication problems by using dimensional analysis. A score of 100%, or all 20 problems answered correctly, is an ideal maximum goal. A score of 80%, or 16 problems answered correctly is a minimum goal. Problems answered incorrectly can be reviewed in the corresponding chapters identified in the Chapter Exercise Answer section until an ideal score of 100% is attained. A score of 100% demonstrates competence and ensures patient safety when calculating a variety of medication problems using dimensional analysis as a problem-solving method.

Comprehensive Post-Test

1. Order: digoxin, 0.125 mg PO daily, for congestive heart failure
   On hand: digoxin 0.25 mg/tablet
   How many tablets will you give?

   Answer: _____

2. Order: ascorbic acid, 0.5 g PO daily, for supplemental therapy
   On hand: ascorbic acid 500 mg/tablet

How many tablets will you give?

Answer: _____

3. Order: atropine, gr 1/150 IM, for on-call preanesthesia
   Supply: atropine 0.4 mg/mL
   How many milliliters will you give?

Answer: _____

4. Order: vancomycin, 2 mg/kg IV every 12 hours, for infection
   Supply: vancomycin 500 mg/10 mL
   Patient's weight: 75 kg
   How many milliliters will you give?

Answer: _____

5. Order: ASA, gr 10 PO every 4 hours, for fever
   On hand: ASA 325 mg/tablet
   How many tablets will you give?

Answer: _____

6. Order: Demerol, 50 mg IM every 4 hours, for pain
   Supply: Demerol 100 mg/mL

How many milliliters will you give?

Answer: ⎯⎯⎯⎯⎯⎯⎯⎯⎯⎯

7. Order: ampicillin, 2 mg/kg PO every 8 hours, for infection
Supply: ampicillin 500 mg/5 mL
Patient's weight: 100 lb
How many milliliters will you give?

Answer: ⎯⎯⎯⎯⎯⎯⎯⎯⎯⎯

8. Order: 1000 mL D5W to infuse in 12 hours
Drop factor: 15 gtt/mL
Calculate the number of drops per minute.

Answer: ⎯⎯⎯⎯⎯⎯⎯⎯⎯⎯

9. Order: 500 mL D5W
Drop factor: 15 gtt/mL
Infusion rate: 21 gtt/min
Calculate hours to infuse.

Answer: ⎯⎯⎯⎯⎯⎯⎯⎯⎯⎯

10. Order: heparin, 1500 units/hr
Supply: 250 mL IV bag of D5W with 25,000 units of heparin

Calculate milliliters per hour to set the IV pump.

Answer: _____

11. Order: dopamine, 4 mcg/kg/min IV, for decreased cardiac output
    Supply: 250 mL D5W with 400 mg of dopamine
    Patient's weight: 120 lb
    Calculate milliliters per hour to set the IV pump.

    Answer: _____

12. Order: Staphcillin, 750 mg IV every 4 hours, for infection
    Supply: Staphcillin 6 g
    Nursing drug reference: Reconstitute with 8 mL of sterile water to yield 1 g/mL.
    How many milliliters will you draw from the vial after reconstitution?

    Answer: _____

13. Order: 1000 mL NS IV
    Drop factor: 15 gtt/mL
    Infusion rate: 50 gtt/min
    Calculate hours to infuse.

    Answer: _____

14. Order: regular insulin, 8 units per hour IV, for hyperglycemia
Supply: 250 mL NS with 100 units of regular insulin
Calculate milliliters per hour to set the IV pump.

Answer: _____

15. Order: Nipride, 0.8 mcg/kg/min IV, for hypertension
Supply: 500 mL D5W with 50 mg Nipride
Patient's weight: 143 lb
Calculate milliliters per hour to set the IV pump.

Answer: _____

16. Order: 500 mL of 10% lipids to infuse in 8 hours
Drop factor: 10 gtt/mL
Calculate the number of drops per minute.

Answer: _____

17. Order: KCl, 2 mEq/100 mL of D5W, for hypokalemia
On hand: 20 mEq/10-mL vial
Supply: 500 mL D5W
How many milliliters of KCl will you add to the IV bag?

Answer: _____

18. Order: Mycostatin oral suspension, 500,000 units swish-and-swallow, for oral thrush
    On hand: Mycostatin 100,000 units/mL
    How many teaspoons will you give?

    Answer: _____

19. Order: aminophylline, 44 mg/hr IV, for bronchodilation
    Supply: 250 mL D5W with 1 g of aminophylline
    Calculate milliliters per hour to set the IV pump.

    Answer: _____

20. Order: Dilaudid, 140 mL/hr
    Supply: 1000 mL D5W/NS with 30 mg of Dilaudid
    Calculate milligrams per hour that the patient is receiving.

    Answer: _____

9

Case Study-Based Clinical Calculations

This chapter presents 10 case studies simulating typical orders that might be written for patients with selected disorders. In each case, the orders include multiple situations that require the nurse to perform clinical calculations before being able to implement the order. After reading the short scenario, read through the list of orders. In the space following each list of orders, write a list of the orders that will require calculations. Then check your list against the list of problems that are set up on the following page. The case scenarios include congestive heart failure, small cell lung cancer, acquired immunodeficiency syndrome (AIDS), sickle cell anemia, deep vein thrombosis, bone marrow transplant, pneumonia, pain, and cirrhosis.

The correct answers to each set of orders requiring calculations are presented at the end of this chapter.

⬭ Case Study A: Congestive Heart Failure

A patient is admitted to the hospital with a diagnosis of dyspnea, peripheral edema with a 10-lb weight gain, and a history of congestive heart failure. The orders from the physician include:

- Bed rest in Fowler's position

- O_2 at 4 L/min per nasal cannula

- Chest x-ray, complete blood count, electrolyte panel, BUN, serum creatinine levels, and a digoxin level

- IV of D5W/$\frac{1}{2}$NS at 50 cc/hr

- Daily AM weight

- Antiembolism stockings

- Furosemide 40 mg IV qd

- Digoxin 0.125 mg PO qd

⊂ **Case Study A** continued

- KCL 20 mEq PO tid

- Low Na diet

- Restrict PO fluids to 1500 cc/day

- Vitals q4h

- Accurate I/O

Identify the orders that will require calculations:

1. _____

2. _____

3. _____

4. _____

5. _____

Set up and solve each problem using dimensional analysis.

1. Calculate gtt/min using a micro tubing (60 gtt/mL).

2. Calculate the weight gain in kilograms.

▭ **Case Study A** continued

3. Calculate how many mL of Lasix the patient will receive IV from a multidose vial labeled 10 mg/mL.

4. Calculate how many tablets of digoxin the patient will receive from a unit dose of 0.25 mg/tablet.

5. Calculate how many tablets of K-Dur the patient will receive from a unit dose of 10 mEq/tablet.

▭ **Case Study B: COPD/emphysema**

A patient is admitted to the hospital with dyspnea and COPD exacerbation. The orders from the physician include:

- Stat ABG's, chest x-ray, complete blood count, and electrolytes
- IV D5W/$\frac{1}{2}$NS 1000 cc/8 hr
- Aminophylline IV loading dose of 5.6 mg/kg over 30 min. followed by 0.5 mg/kg/hr continuous IV
- O_2 at 2L/min per nasal cannula
- Albuterol respiratory treatments q4h
- Chest physiotherapy q4h
- Erythromycin 800 mg IV q6h
- Bed rest
- Accurate I/O

◯ **Case Study B** continued

- High-calorie, protein-rich diet in 6 small meals daily

- Encourage PO fluids to 3L/day

Identify the orders that will require calculations:

1. _____

2. _____

3. _____

4. _____

5. _____

Set up and solve each problem using dimensional analysis.

1. Calculate cc/hr to set the IV pump.

2. Calculate cc/hr to set the IV pump for the loading dose of aminophylline for a patient weighing 140 lb. Aminophylline supply: 100 mg/100 mL D5W.

○ **Case Study B** continued

3. Calculate cc/hr to set the IV pump for the continuous dose of aminophylline for a patient weighing 140 lb. Aminophylline supply: 1 gm/250 mL D$_5$W.

4. Calculate cc/hr to set the IV pump to infuse erythromycin 800 mg. Erythromycin supply: 1-gm vial to be reconstituted with 20 cc sterile water and further diluted in 250 cc NS to infuse over 1 hr.

5. Calculate the PO fluids in cc/shift.

○ **Case Study C: Small Cell Lung Cancer**

A patient with small cell lung cancer is admitted to the hospital with fever and dehydration. The orders from the physician include:

- O$_2$ at 2L/min per nasal cannula

- Chest x-ray, complete blood count, electrolytes, blood, urine, and sputum cultures, BUN and serum creatinine levels, type and cross for 2 units of PRBC's

- IV D5W/$\frac{1}{2}$NS 1000 cc with 10 mEq KCL at 125 cc/hr

- 2 units of PBRC's if Hg is below 8

- 6 pack of platelets if <20,000

- Neupogen 5 mcg/kg SQ daily

- Gentamicin 80 mg IV q8h

- Decadron 8 mg IV daily

- Fortaz 1 gm IV q8hr

◯ **Case Study C** continued

- Accurate I/O

- Encourage PO fluids

- Vitals q4h (call for temperature > 102°F)

Identify the orders that will require calculations:

1. ————————————————

2. ————————————————

3. ————————————————

4. ————————————————

5. ————————————————

Set up and solve each problem using dimensional analysis.

1. Calculate gtt/min using a macro tubing (20 gtt/mL).

2. Calculate how many mcg of Neupogen will be given SQ to a patient weighing 160 lb.

⊂ **Case Study C** continued

3. Calculate cc/hr to set the IV pump to infuse Gentamicin. The vial is labeled 40 mg/mL and is to be further diluted in 100 cc D5W to infuse over 1 hr.

4. Calculate how many ml of Decadron the patient will receive from a vial labeled Dexamethasone 4 mg/mL.

5. Calculate cc/hr to set the IV pump to infuse Fortaz 1 gm over 30 minutes. Supply: Fortaz 1 gm/50 mL.

⊂ **Case Study D: Acquired Immunodeficiency Syndrome (AIDS)**

A patient who is HIV+ and a Jehovah's Witness is admitted to the hospital with anemia, fever of unknown origin, and wasting syndrome with dehydration. The orders from the physician include:

- O_2 at 4L/min per nasal cannula
- IV D5W/$\frac{1}{2}$NS at 150 cc/hr
- CD4 and CD8 T-cell subset counts, erythrocyte sedimentation rate, complete blood count, urine, sputum, and stool cultures, chest x-ray
- Acyclovir 350 mg IV q8h
- Neupogen 300 mcg SQ daily
- Epogen 100 units/kg SQ 3 times a week
- Megace 40 mg PO tid

◻ **Case Study D** continued

- Zidovudine 100 mg PO q4h

- Vancomycin 800 mg IV q6h

- Respiratory treatments with pentamidine

- High-calorie, protein-rich diet in 6 small meals daily

- Encourage PO fluids to 3L/day

- Accurate I/O

- Daily AM weight

Identify the orders that will require calculations:

1. _____

2. _____

3. _____

4. _____

5. _____

Set up and solve each problem using dimensional analysis.

1. Calculate gtt/min using a macro tubing (20 gtt/mL).

▭ **Case Study D** continued

2. Calculate cc/hr to set the IV pump to infuse acyclovir 350 mg. Supply: 500-mg vial to be reconstituted with 10 mL sterile water and further diluted in 100 ml D5W to infuse over 1 hr.

3. Calculate how many mL of Neupogen will be given SQ. The vial is labeled 300 mcg/mL.

4. Calculate how many ml of Epogen will be given SQ to the patient weighing 100 lb. The vial is labeled 4,000 units/mL.

5. Calculate how many cc/hr to set the IV pump to infuse vancomycin 800 mg. Supply: 1-gm vials to be reconstituted with 10 mL NS and further diluted in 100 mL D5W to infuse over 60 min.

▭ **Case Study E: Sickle Cell Anemia**

A patient is admitted to the hospital in sickle cell crisis. The orders from the physician include:

- Bed rest with joint support
- O_2 at 2L/min per nasal cannula
- Complete blood count, erythrocyte sedimentation rate, serum iron levels, and chest x-ray
- IV D5W/$\frac{1}{2}$NS at 150 cc/hr
- Zofran 8 mg IV q8h

◯ **Case Study E** continued

- Morphine sulfate 5 mg IV PRN

- Hydrea 10 mg/kg/day PO

- Folic acid 0.5 mg daily PO

- Encourage 3000 cc/daily PO

Identify the orders that will require calculations:

1. _____

2. _____

3. _____

4. _____

5. _____

Set up and solve each problem using dimensional analysis.

1. Calculate gtt/min using a macro tubing (10 gtt/mL).

2. Calculate cc/hr to set the IV pump to infuse Zofran 8 mg. Supply: Zofran 8 mg in 50 cc D5W to infuse over 15 min.

○ **Case Study E** continued

3. Calculate how many ml of morphine sulfate will be given IV. The syringe is labeled 10 mg/mL.

4. Calculate how many mg/day of Hydrea will be given PO to the patient weighing 125 lb.

5. Calculate how many tablets of folic acid will be given PO. Supply: 1 mg/tablet.

○ **Case Study F: Deep Vein Thombosis**

A patient is admitted to the hospital with right leg erythema and edema to R/O DVT. The orders from the physician include:

- Bed rest with right leg elevated

- Warm, moist heat to right leg with Aqua-K pad

- Doppler ultrasonography

- Partial thromboplastin time (PTT) and prothrombin time (PT)

- IV D5W/$\frac{1}{2}$NS with 20 mEq KCL at 50 cc/hr

- Heparin 5000 units IV Push followed by continuous IV infusion of 1000 units/hr

- Lasix 20 mg IV bid

- Morphine 5 mg IV q4h

⊂ **Case Study F** continued

Identify the orders that will require calculations:

1. _____

2. _____

3. _____

4. _____

5. _____

Set up and solve each problem using dimensional analysis.

1. Calculate gtt/min using a macro tubing (60 gtt/mL).

2. Calculate how many mL of heparin the patient will receive IV from a multidose vial labeled 10,000 units/mL.

3. Calculate cc/hr to set the IV pump for the continuous dose of heparin. Heparin supply: 25,000 units/250 mL D5W.

◯ **Case Study F** continued

4. Calculate how many ml of Lasix the patient will receive IV from a multidose vial labeled 10 mg/mL.

5. Calculate how many ml of morphine the patient will receive from a syringe labeled 10 mg/mL.

◯ **Case Study G: Bone Marrow Transplant**

A patient is admitted to the hospital with a rash following an allogeneic bone marrow transplant. The orders from the physician include:

- IV D5W/$\frac{1}{2}$NS with 20 mEq KCL/L at 80 cc/hr
- Complete blood count, electrolytes, culture sputum, urine, and stool, blood cultures ×3, liver panel, BUN, and creatinine
- Vitals q4h
- Strict I/O
- Fortaz 2 gm IV q 8h
- Vancomycin 1 gm IV q 6h
- Claforan 1 gm IV q 12h
- Erythromycin 800 mg IV q6h

Identify the orders that will require calculations:

1. _____

◯ **Case Study G** continued

2. _____

3. _____

4. _____

5. _____

Set up and solve each problem using dimensional analysis.

1. Calculate how many mEq per hr of KCL the patient will receive IV.

2. Calculate cc/hr to set the IV pump to infuse Fortaz 2 gm. Supply: Fortaz 2-gm vial to be reconstituted with 10 mL of sterile water and further diluted in 50 cc D5W to infuse over 30 min.

3. Calculate cc/hr to set the IV pump to infuse vancomycin 1 gm. Supply: vancomycin 500-mg vial to be reconstituted with 10 mL of sterile water and further diluted in 100 mL of D5W to infuse over 60 min.

4. Calculate cc/hr to set the IV pump to infuse Claforan 1 gm. Supply: Claforan 600 mg/4 mL to be further diluted with 100 cc D5W to infuse over 1 hr.

⊙ **Case Study G** continued

5. Calculate cc/hr to set the IV pump to infuse erythromycin 800 mg. Supply: Erythromycin 1-gm vial to be diluted with 20 mL sterile water and further diluted in 250 mL of NS to infuse over 60 min.

⊙ **Case Study H: Pneumonia**

A patient is admitted to the hospital with fever, cough, chills, and dyspnea to rule out pneumonia. The orders from the physician include:

- IV 600 cc D5W q8h

- I/O

- Vitals q4h

- Complete blood count, electrolytes, chest x-ray, ABG's, sputum specimen, blood cultures, and bronchoscopy

- Bed rest

- Humidified O_2 at 4L/min per nasal cannula

- High-calorie diet

- Encourage oral fluids of 2000–3000 mL/day

- Pulse oximetry qAM

- Clindamycin 400 mg IV q 6h

- Albuterol respiratory treatments

- Guaifenesin 200 mg PO q4h

- Terbutaline 2.5 mg PO TID

- MS Contrin 30 mg PO q4h prn

◯ **Case Study H** continued

Identify the orders that will require calculations:

1. _____

2. _____

3. _____

4. _____

5. _____

Set up and solve each problem using dimensional analysis.

1. Calculate cc/hr to set the IV pump to infuse clindamycin 400 mg. Supply: Clindamycin 600 mg/4 mL to be further diluted with 50 mL D5W to infuse over 1 hr.

2. Calculate gtt/min to infuse the clindamycin using a macro tubing (20gtt/mL).

3. Calculate how many cc of guaifenesin the patient will receive from a stock bottle labeled 30 mg/tsp.

⊂ **Case Study H** continued

4. Calculate how many tablets of terbutaline the patient will receive from a unit dose of 5 mg/tablet.

5. Calculate how many tablets of MS Contrin the patient will receive from a unit dose of 30 mg/tablet.

⊂ **Case Study I: Pain**

A patient is admitted to the hospital with intractable bone pain secondary to prostate cancer. The orders from the physician include:

- IV D5W/$\frac{1}{2}$NS with 20 mEq KCL/L at 60 cc/hr

- IV 500 cc NS with 25 mg Dilaudid and 50 mg Thorazine at 21 cc/hr

- Heparin 25,000 units/250 cc D5W at 11 cc/hr

- Bed rest

- Do not resuscitate

- O_2 at 2L/min per nasal cannula

- Bumex 2 mg IV qAM following albumin infusion

- Albumin 12.5 gm IV qAM

Identify the orders that will require calculations:

1. _____

○ **Case Study I** continued

2. _____

3. _____

4. _____

5. _____

Set up and solve each problem using dimensional analysis.

1. Calculate how many mEq/hr of KCL the patient is receiving.

2. Calculate how many mg/hr of Dilaudid the patient is receiving.

3. Calculate how many mg/hr of Thorazine the patient is receiving.

4. Calculate how many units/hr of heparin the patient is receiving.

○ **Case Study I** continued

5. Calculate how many cc of Bumex the patient will receive from a stock dose of 0.25 mg/mL.

○ **Case Study J: Cirrhosis**

A patient is admitted to the hospital with ascites, stomach pain, and dyspnea and a history of cirrhosis of the liver. The orders from the physician include:

- IV D5W/$\frac{1}{2}$NS with 20 mEq KCL at 125 cc/hr

- IV Zantac 150 mg/250 cc NS at 11 cc/hr

- O_2 at 2L/min per nasal cannula

- Type and cross match for 2 units of packed red blood cells, complete blood count, liver panel, PT/PTT, SMA-12.

- Carafate 1 gm q4h

- Vitamin K 10 mg SQ qAM

- Spironolactone 50 mg PO BID

- Lasix 80 mg IV qAM

- Measure abdominal girth qAM

- Sodium restriction to 500 mg/day

- Fluid restriction to 1500 cc/day

Identify the orders that will require calculations:

1. _____

2. _____

○ **Case Study J** continued

3. _____

4. _____

5. _____

Set up and solve each problem using dimensional analysis.

1. Calculate the gtt/min using a macro tubing (20 gtt/mL).

2. Calculate the mg/hr of Zantac the patient is receiving.

3. Calculate how many cc of vitamin K the patient will receive SQ from a unit dose labeled 10 mg/mL.

4. Calculate how many tablets of spironolactone the patient will receive from a unit dose labeled 25 mg/tablet.

5. Calculate how many cc of Lasix the patient will receive from a unit dose labeled 10 mg/mL.

Appendix

Contents

A. Containers Used to Administer Oral Medications
   Medicine Cup
   Medication Syringe
B. Types of Syringes
   Insulin Syringes
   Tuberculin Syringe
   3 cc Syringe
C. Abbreviations
D. Systems of Measurement
   Metric Weights
   Metric Volume
   Apothecary Weights
   Apothecary Volume
   Household
E. Approximate Equivalents Among the Metric, Apothecary and Household Systems
F. Quick Summary of Dimensional Analysis Terms, Steps and Unit Path

⊂⊃ APPENDIX A

CONTAINERS USED TO ADMINISTER ORAL MEDICATIONS

Medicine Cup

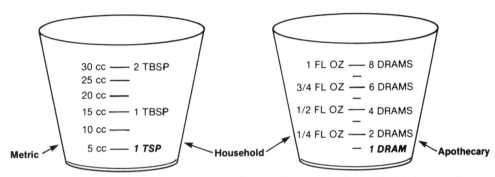

A medicine cup for measurement of metric, apothecary, or household dose units.

Medication Syringe

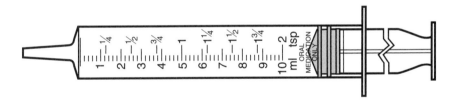

⬭ APPENDIX B

TYPES OF SYRINGES

Insulin Syringes

A 0.5-mL (cc) low-dose insulin syringe for U 100 insulin.

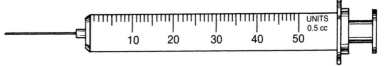

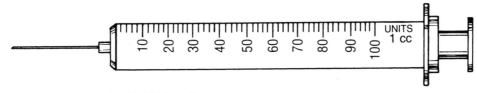

A 1-mL (cc) insulin syringe for U 100 insulin.

Tuberculin Syringe

A 1-mL (cc) precision syringe with metric and apothecary measures.

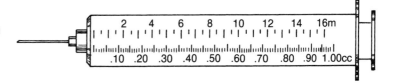

3 cc Syringe

A 3-mL (cc) syringe with metric and apothecary measures.

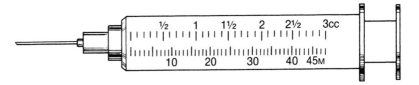

○ APPENDIX C

ABBREVIATIONS

$\bar{a}$ or a	before		L	liter
ac	before meals		lb	pound
ad lib	as desired, freely		liq	liquid
AM	in the morning, before noon		m	meter
bid	twice a day		M or M̧	minim
$\bar{c}$	with		mcg	microgram
cap or caps	capsule		mEq	milliequivalent
cc	cubic centimeter		mg	milligram
cm	centimeter		min	minute
dr or ʒ	dram		ml	milliliter
DC	discontinue		NPO	nothing by mouth
DX	diagnosis		NS	normal saline, sodium chloride or 0.9% NS
D5W	Dextrose 5% in Water			
D5/$\frac{1}{2}$NS	Dextrose 5% in Water with $\frac{1}{2}$ Normal Saline		OD	right eye
			OS	left eye
elix	elixir		os	mouth
et	and		oz or ʒ	ounce
fl or fld	fluid		OU	both eyes
g or gm	gram		$\bar{p}$	after
gal	gallon		p	per
gr	grain		PB	piggyback
gtt	drop		pc	after meals
h or hr	hour		per	by
hs	hour of sleep (bedtime)		po or per os	by mouth
IM	intramuscular(ly)		PM	afternoon or evening
inj	injection		prn	as needed or when necessary
iss	$1\frac{1}{2}$ or one and a half		pt	pint
IV	intravenous(ly)		q	every
IVPB	intravenous piggyback		qd	every day
kg	kilogram		qh	every hour
KCL	potassium chloride		q2h	every 2 hours
KVO	keep vein open		q3h	every 3 hours

○ **APPENDIX C** continued

ABBREVIATIONS

q4h	every 4 hours	**SL**	sublingual (beneath the tongue)
q6h	every 6 hours	**SQ**	subcutaneous(ly)
q8h	every 8 hours	**s̄s**	$\frac{1}{2}$ or half
qid	four times a day	**stat**	immediately or at once
qod	every other day	**supp**	suppository
qt	quart	**tab**	tablet
R	rectal	**tbs, tbsp, T**	tablespoon
R/O	rule out	**tid**	three times a day
RX	treatment	**TKO**	to keep open
s̄	without	**tsp, t**	teaspoon
SC	subcutaneous(ly)	**U**	unit

⬭ APPENDIX D

SYSTEMS OF MEASUREMENT

> **Metric System Units of Weight and Equivalents**
>
> 1 kilogram (kg)
> 1 gram (g)
> 1 milligram (mg)
> 1 microgram (mcg)
> 1 kg = 1000 g
> 1 g = 1000 mg
> 1 mg = 1000 mcg

> **Metric System Units of Volume and Equivalents**
>
> 1 liter (L)
> 1 milliliter (mL)
> 1 cubic centimeter (cc)
> 1 L = 1000 mL
> 1 mL = 1 cc

> **Apothecary System Units of Weight and Equivalents**
>
> 1 pound (lb)
> 1 ounce (oz)
> 1 dram (dr)
> 1 grain (gr)
> 1 lb = 16 oz
> 1 oz = 8 dr
> 1 dr = 60 gr

Apothecary System Unit of Volume and Equivalents

1 gallon (gal)
1 quart (qt)
1 pint (pt)
1 fluid ounce (foz)
1 fluid dram (fdr)
1 minim (M)
1 gal = 4 qt
1 qt = 2 pt
1 pt = 16 foz
1 foz = 8 fdr
1 fdr = 60 M
1 foz = 1 oz
1 fdr = 1 dr

Household Measurement System and Equivalents

1 glass
1 cup
1 tablespoon (tbsp or T)
1 teaspoon (tsp or t)
1 drop (gtt)
1 glass = 8 ounces (oz)
1 cup = 6 ounces (oz)
2 Tbsp = 1 oz
3 tsp = 1 tbsp
1 tsp = 60 gtt

○ APPENDIX E

Approximate Equivalents

Metric	Apothecary	Household
1 kg = 1000 g	= 2.2 lb	
	1 lb = 16 oz	
1 g = 1000 mg	= 15 gr	
60 mg	= 1 gr	
1 mg = 1000 mcg		
4000 mL	= 1 gal = 4 qt	
1 L = 1000 mL	= 1 qt = 2 pt	
500 mL	= 1 pt = 16 foz	
240 cc	= 8 oz	= 1 glass
180 cc	= 6 oz	= 1 cup
30 cc	= 1 oz = 8 dr	= 2 tbsp
15 cc	= $\frac{1}{2}$ oz = 4 dr	= 1 tbsp = 3 tsp
5 cc	= 1 dr = 60 M	= 1 tsp = 60 gtt
1 mL = 1 cc	= 15 M	= 15 gtts
	1 M	= 1 gtt

◯ APPENDIX F

DIMENSIONAL ANALYSIS TERMS:
- GIVEN QUANTITY—the beginning point of the problem.

- WANTED QUANTITY—the answer to the problem.

- UNIT PATH—the series of conversions necessary to achieve the answer to the problem.

- CONVERSION FACTORS—equivalents necessary to convert between systems of measurement and allow unwanted united to be canceled from the problem.

THE FIVE STEPS OF DIMENSIONAL ANALYSIS:
1. Identify the *given quantity* in the problem.

2. Identify the *wanted quantity* in the problem.

3. Establish the *unit path* from the *given quantity* to the *wanted quantity* using equivalents as *conversion factors.*

4. Set up the problem to allow for cancellation of unwanted units.

5. Multiply the numerators, multiply the denominators and divide the product of the numerators by the product of the denominators to provide the numerical value of the *wanted quantity.*

Below is an example of the problem-solving method, showing the placement of basic terms used in dimensional analysis.

Unit Path

Given Quantity	Conversion Factor For Given Quantity	Conversion Factor For Wanted Quantity	Conversion Computation		Wanted Quantity
1 liter (~~L~~)	1000 ~~mL~~	1 (oz)	1 × 1000 × 1 oz	1000	= 33.3 ounces
	1 liter (~~L~~)	30 ~~mL~~	1 × 30	30	

BIBLIOGRAPHY

Bevis, E. (1988). New directions for a new age. In National League for Nursing, *Curriculum revolution: Mandate for change* (pp. 27–52). New York: National League for Nursing (Pub. No. 15-2224).

Bruner, J. (1960). *The process of education.* New York: Random House.

Craig, G. (1995). The effects of dimensional analysis on the medication dosage calculation abilities of nursing students. *Nurse Educator, 20*(3), 14–18.

Goodstein, M. (1983). Reflections upon mathematics in the introductory chemistry course. *Journal of Chemical Education, 60*(8), 665–667.

Hein, M. (1983). *Foundations of chemistry* (4th ed.). Encino, CA: Dickenson Publishing Company.

Lindeman, C. (1989). Curriculum revolution: Reconceptualizing clinical nursing education. *Nursing and Health Care, 10*(1), 23–28.

National Institute of Education. (1984). *Involvement in learning: Realizing the potential of American higher education.* Washington DC: National Institute of Education.

Peters, E. (1986). *Introduction to chemical principles* (4th ed.). Saratoga, CA: Saunders College Publishing.

Tanner, C. (1988). Curriculum revolution: The practice mandate. *Nursing and Health Care, 9*(8), 426–430.

GLOSSARY

Apothecary System: a system of measuring and weighing drugs and solutions in which fractions are used to identify parts of the unit of measure. The basic units of measurement include weights and liquid volume.

Conversion Factors: equivalents necessary to convert between systems of measurement and allow unwanted units to be canceled from the problem.

Denominator: the number on the bottom portion of the fraction that represents the number of parts into which the whole is divided.

Digits: symbols used in the Arabic number system.

Diluent: a specific amount of sterile solution used to reconstitute medications.

Dimensional Analysis: a problem-solving method that can be used whenever two quantities are directly proportional to each other and one quantity must be converted to the other using a common equivalent, conversion factor, or conversion relationship.

Dividing Line: the line separating the top portion of the fraction from the bottom portion of the fraction.

Drop Factor: the number of drops per milliliter (gtt/mL) that intravenous tubing will deliver, including **macro** (tubing that delivers large drops and is available in 10 gtt/mL, 15 gtt/mL, and 20 gtt/mL) and **micro** (tubing that delivers small drops and is available in 60 gtt/mL).

Drug Label: the label on stock or unit-dose medication that contains specific information to assist in the accurate administration of the medication.

Enteric-Coated: tablets that have a special external coating that prevents the release of medication in the stomach and thereby decreases irritation, and dissolves later in the small intestine for absorption.

Factor in or Factored into: incorporating information or conversion factors into the problem.

Five Rights: the information necessary for accurate medication administration, including the right drug, the right dose, the right route, the right time, and the right patient.

Fraction: a number that represents a part of a whole number and contains three parts, including a numerator, a dividing line, and a denominator.

201

Given Quantity: the beginning point of the problem.

Gravity Flow: intravenous fluids or medications that are administered without an IV pump and require calculation of drops per minute (gtt/min) to administer.

Household Measurements: the use of measuring devices in the home, including cups, glasses, and eating utensils.

Intermittent Infusion: intravenous fluids or medications that must be delivered over a specific amount of time.

Metric System: a decimal system of weights and measure based on units of ten in which gram, meter, and liter are the basic units of measurement.

Numerator: the number on the top portion of the fraction that represents the number of parts of the whole fraction.

One-Factor Medication Problems: medication problems that contain only numerators in the given quantity or the wanted quantity portion of the medication problem.

Parenteral: medications delivered by subcutaneous (SQ), intramuscular (IM), or intravenous (IV) administration.

Random Method: a dimensional analysis problemsolving method that focuses on the correct placement of conversion factors to correlate with the wanted quantity in the numerator portion of the unit path without consideration of preceding units.

Reconstitution: adding a specific amount of sterile solution to a vial of medication to dissolve a powder into a liquid form.

Scored Tablets: a tablet that can be cut in half, allowing the exact dosage of medication to be administered.

Sequential Method: a dimensional analysis problem-solving method that focuses on the correct placement of conversion factors to cancel out the preceding unit.

Symbols: a graphic representation of a number in the Roman numeral system.

Three-Factor Medication Problems: medication problems that contain three parts, including a numerator (the dosage of medication ordered) and two denominators (the weight of the patient and the time required for safe administration) in the given quantity or wanted quantity portion of the medication problem.

Time-Released: medication in capsule form that is released into the system over a specific amount of time.

Titrate: an increase or decrease in intravenous fluids or medications based on the effectiveness experienced by the patient.

Two-Factor Medication Problems: medication problems that contain a numerator and a denominator in the given quantity or the wanted quantity portion of the medication problem.

Unit Path: the series of conversions necessary to achieve the answer to the problem.

Wanted Quantity: the answer to the problem.

Yield: the amount of medication per milliliter that is produced after adding a specific amount of sterile solution to a vial to dissolve a powder into a liquid form.

CHAPTER EXERCISE ANSWERS

CHAPTER 1

Exercise 1

1.	1	= I
2.	1 + 1	= II
3.	1 + 1 + 1	= III
4.	5 − 1	= IV
5.	5	= V
6.	5 + 1	= VI
7.	5 + 1 + 1	= VII
8.	5 + 1 + 1 + 1	= VIII
9.	10 − 1	= IX
10.	10	= X
11.	10 + 1	= XI
12.	10 + 1 + 1	= XII
13.	10 + 1 + 1 + 1	= XIII
14.	10 + 5 − 1	= XIV
15.	10 + 5	= XV
16.	10 + 5 + 1	= XVI
17.	10 + 5 + 1 + 1	= XVII
18.	10 + 5 + 1 + 1	= XVIII
19.	10 + 10 − 1	= XIX
20.	10 + 10	= XX

Exercise 2

1.	50 − 10 + 1 + 1 + 1	= XLIII
2.	10 + 10 + 5 − 1	= XXIV
3.	50 + 5	= LV
4.	10 + 10 + 10 + 1 + 1	= XXXII

○ **Chapter 1** continued

```
 5.  100 + 1 + 1            = CII
 6.  100 + 50               = CL
 7.  50 + 10 + 10 + 5       = LXXV
 8.  100 − 10 + 1 + 1       = XCII
 9.  50 + 10 + 5 − 1        = LXIV
10.  50 + 10 + 10 − 1       = LXIX
```

Exercise 3

```
 1.  1 + 1                 = 2
 2.  5 − 1                 = 4
 3.  5 + 1                 = 6
 4.  10                    = 10
 5.  5 + 1 + 1 + 1         = 8
 6.  10 − 1 + 10           = 19
 7.  10 + 10               = 20
 8.  10 + 5 + 1 + 1 + 1    = 18
 9.  1                     = 1
10.  10 + 5                = 15
11.  1 + 1 + 1             = 3
12.  5                     = 5
13.  10 − 1                = 9
14.  5 + 1 + 1             = 7
15.  10 + 1                = 11
16.  10 + 5 − 1            = 14
17.  10 + 5 + 1            = 16
18.  10 + 1 + 1            = 12
19.  10 + 5 + 1 + 1        = 17
20.  10 + 1 + 1 + 1        = 13
```

Exercise 4

```
1.  19   = XIX
2.  XII  = 12
3.  7    = VII
4.  IX   = 9
5.  IV   = 4
6.  11   = XI
7.  VIII = 8
8.  16   = XVI
9.  XX   = 20
```

10. 5   = V
11. I   = 1
12. 18 = XVIII
13. VI = 6
14. 2   = II
15. III = 3
16. 10 = X
17. XIII = 13
18. 14 = XIV
19. XV = 15
20. 17 = XVII

Exercise 5

1. 34   = XXXIV
2. XXII = 22
3. 75   = LXXV
4. XC   = 90
5. 29   = XXIX
6. XLII = 42
7. 56   = LVI
8. LXIV = 64
9. 88   = LXXXVIII
10. CXXI = 121

Exercise 6

1. $\frac{3}{4} \times \frac{5}{8} = \frac{3 \times 5 = 15}{4 \times 8 = 32} = \frac{15}{32}$

2. $\frac{1}{3} \times \frac{4}{9} = \frac{1 \times 4 = 4}{3 \times 9 = 27} = \frac{4}{27}$

3. $\frac{2}{3} \times \frac{4}{5} = \frac{2 \times 4 = 8}{3 \times 5 = 15} = \frac{8}{15}$

4. $\frac{3}{4} \times \frac{1}{2} = \frac{3 \times 1 = 3}{4 \times 2 = 8} = \frac{3}{8}$

5. $\frac{1}{8} \times \frac{4}{5} = \frac{1 \times 4 = 4(4) = 1}{8 \times 5 = 40(4) = 10} = \frac{1}{10}$

6. $\frac{2}{3} \times \frac{5}{8} = \frac{2 \times 5 = 10(2) = 5}{3 \times 8 = 24(2) = 12} = \frac{5}{12}$

7. $\frac{3}{8} \times \frac{2}{3} = \frac{3 \times 2 = 6(6) = 1}{8 \times 3 = 24(6) = 4} = \frac{1}{4}$

8. $\frac{4}{7} \times \frac{2}{4} = \frac{4 \times 2 = 8(4) = 2}{7 \times 4 = 28(4) = 7} = \frac{2}{7}$

9. $\frac{4}{5} \times \frac{1}{2} = \frac{4 \times 1 = 4(2) = 2}{5 \times 2 = 10(2) = 5} = \frac{2}{5}$

10. $\frac{1}{4} \times \frac{1}{8} = \frac{1 \times 1 = 1}{4 \times 8 = 32} = \frac{1}{32}$

⚪ **Chapter 1** continued

Exercise 7

1. $\frac{3}{4} \div \frac{2}{3} = \frac{3}{4} \times \frac{3}{2}$ or $\frac{3 \times 3 = 9}{4 \times 2 = 8} = 8\overline{)9}^{\,1\frac{1}{8}} = 1\frac{1}{8}$
$$\underline{8}$$
$$1$$

2. $\frac{1}{9} \div \frac{3}{9} = \frac{1}{9} \times \frac{9}{3}$ or $\frac{1 \times 9 = 9\,(9) = 1}{9 \times 3 = 27(9) = 3} = \frac{1}{3}$

3. $\frac{2}{3} \div \frac{1}{6} = \frac{2}{3} \times \frac{6}{1}$ or $\frac{2 \times 6 = 12}{3 \times 1 = 3} = 3\overline{)12}^{\,4} = 4$
$$\underline{12}$$

4. $\frac{1}{5} \div \frac{4}{5} = \frac{1}{5} \times \frac{5}{4}$ or $\frac{1 \times 5 = 5\,(5) = 1}{5 \times 4 = 20(5) = 4} = \frac{1}{4}$

5. $\frac{3}{6} \div \frac{4}{8} = \frac{3}{6} \times \frac{8}{4}$ or $\frac{3 \times 8 = 24}{6 \times 4 = 24} = 24\overline{)24}^{\,1} = 1$

6. $\frac{5}{8} \div \frac{5}{8} = \frac{5}{8} \times \frac{8}{5}$ or $\frac{5 \times 8 = 40}{8 \times 5 = 40} = 40\overline{)40}^{\,1} = 1$

7. $\frac{1}{8} \div \frac{2}{3} = \frac{1}{8} \times \frac{3}{2}$ or $\frac{1 \times 3 = 3}{8 \times 2 = 16} = \frac{3}{16}$

8. $\frac{1}{5} \div \frac{1}{2} = \frac{1}{5} \times \frac{2}{1}$ or $\frac{1 \times 2 = 2}{5 \times 1 = 5} = \frac{2}{5}$

Exercise 8

1. $\frac{1}{8} = 0.125$

$$
\begin{array}{r}
0.125 \\
8\overline{)1.000} \\
\underline{8} \\
20 \\
\underline{16} \\
40 \\
\underline{40} \\
0
\end{array}
$$

Answer = 0.125

2. $\frac{1}{4} = 0.25$

$$
\begin{array}{r}
.25 \\
4\overline{)1.00} \\
\underline{8} \\
20 \\
\underline{20} \\
0
\end{array}
$$

Answer = 0.25

3. $\frac{2}{5} = 0.4$

$$
\begin{array}{r}
0.4 \\
5\overline{)2.0} \\
\underline{2\ 0} \\
0
\end{array}
$$

Answer = 0.4

4. $\frac{3}{5} = 0.6$

$$
\begin{array}{r}
0.6 \\
5\overline{)3.0} \\
\underline{3\ 0} \\
0
\end{array}
$$

Answer = 0.6

5. $\frac{2}{3} = 0.66$

$$
\begin{array}{r}
0.66 \\
3\overline{)2.00} \\
\underline{1\ 8} \\
20 \\
\underline{18} \\
2
\end{array}
$$

Answer = 0.66

◯ **Chapter 1** continued

6. $\frac{6}{8} = 0.75$

$$
\begin{array}{r}
0.75 \\
8\overline{)6.00} \\
\underline{5\ 6} \\
40 \\
\underline{40} \\
0
\end{array}
$$

Answer = 0.75

7. $\frac{3}{8} = 0.375$

$$
\begin{array}{r}
.375 \\
8\overline{)3.000} \\
\underline{2\ 4} \\
60 \\
\underline{56} \\
40 \\
\underline{40} \\
0
\end{array}
$$

Answer = 0.75

8. $\frac{1}{3} = 0.33$

$$
\begin{array}{r}
0.33 \\
3\overline{)1.00} \\
\underline{9} \\
10 \\
\underline{9} \\
1
\end{array}
$$

Answer = 0.33

9. $\frac{3}{6} = 0.5$

$$
\begin{array}{r}
0.5 \\
6\overline{)3.0} \\
\underline{3\ 0} \\
0
\end{array}
$$

Answer = 0.5

10. $\frac{2}{10} = 0.2$

$$
\begin{array}{r}
0.2 \\
10\overline{)2.0} \\
\underline{2\ 0} \\
0
\end{array}
$$

Answer = 0.2

Exercise 9

1. 0.75 = 0.8
2. 0.88 = 0.9
3. 0.44 = 0.4
4. 0.23 = 0.2
5. 0.67 = 0.7
6. 0.27 = 0.3
7. 0.98 = 1.0
8. 0.92 = 0.9

Exercise 10

1. $\quad$ 2.5 (1 decimal point)
    $\times \underline{4.6}$ (1 decimal point)
    $\overline{150}$
    $\underline{1000}$
    $\overline{1150}$
    11.50 (2 decimal points from the right to left)

2. $\quad$ 1.45 (2 decimal points)
    $\times \underline{0.25}$ (2 decimal points)
    $\overline{725}$
    2900
    $\underline{0000}$
    $\overline{3625}$
    0.3625 (4 decimal points from the right to left)

3. $\quad$ 3.9 (1 decimal point)
    $\times \underline{0.8}$ (1 decimal point)
    $\overline{312}$
    $\underline{000}$
    $\overline{312}$
    3.12 (2 decimal points from the right to left)

○ **Chapter 1** continued

4.   2.56 (2 decimal points)
     ×0.45 (2 decimal points)
      1280
    10240
    00000
    11520
   1.1520 (4 decimal points from the right to left)

5.   10.65 (2 decimal points)
    ×0.05 (2 decimal points)
     5325
     0000
     5325
   0.5325 (4 decimal points from the right to left)

6.   1.98 (2 decimal points)
     ×3.10 (2 decimal points)
      000
     1980
    59400
    61380
   6.1380 (4 decimal points from the right to left)

Exercise 11

1. 3.4)$\overline{9.6}$

   (Move decimal points one place to the right)

   Answer: 2.82 = 2.8

```
        2.82
   34)96.00
      68
      ----
      28 0
      27 2
      -----
         80
         68
         ---
         12
```

2. 0.25)$\overline{12.50}$

   (Move decimal points two places to the right)

Answer: 50. = 50

```
        50.
  25)1250.
     125
      00
```

3. 0.56)18.65

(Move decimal points two places to the right)

Answer: 33.30 = 33.3

```
        33.30
  56)1865.00
     168
     185
     168
      17 0
      16 8
         20
```

4. 0.3)0.192

(Move decimal points one place to the right)

Answer: 0.64 = 0.6

```
      .64
  3)01.92
    1 8
     12
     12
      0
```

5. 0.4)12.43

(Move decimal points one place to the right)

Answer: 31.075 = 31.1

○ **Chapter 1** continued

```
        31.075
    4)124.300
      12
      ‾‾
      04
       4
      ‾‾
      0 30
        28
        ‾‾
        20
        20
        ‾‾
         0
```

6. 0.5)12.50

   (Move decimal points one place to the right)

   Answer: 25.0 = 25

```
        25.0
    5)125.0
      10
      ‾‾
      25
      25
      ‾‾
       0
```

7. 0.125)0.25

   (Move decimal points three places to the right)

   Answer: 2. = 2

```
           2
    125)250
        250
        ‾‾‾
          0
```

8. 0.08)0.085

   (Move decimal points two places to the right)

   Answer: 1.0625 = 1.1

```
      1.0625
  8)8.5000
    8
    ‾‾
    50
    48
    ‾‾
    20
    16
    ‾‾
    40
    40
    ‾‾
     0
```

Practice Problems

1. II

2. IV

3. V

4. XIV

5. XIX

6. 6

7. 9

8. 12

9. 17

10. 19

11. $\dfrac{3 \times 2 = 6\,(2) = 3}{4 \times 5 = 20(2) = 10} = \dfrac{3}{10}$

12. $\dfrac{2 \times 5 = 10(2) = 5}{3 \times 8 = 24(2) = 12} = \dfrac{5}{12}$

13. $\dfrac{1 \times 2 = 2(2) = 1}{2 \times 3 = 6(2) = 3} = \dfrac{1}{3}$

14. $\dfrac{7 \times 1 = 7}{8 \times 3 = 24} = \dfrac{7}{24}$

⬭ **Chapter 1** continued

15. $\dfrac{4 \times 2 = 8}{5 \times 7 = 35} = \dfrac{8}{35}$

16. $\dfrac{1}{2} \div \dfrac{3}{4} = \dfrac{1 \times 4 = 4(2) = 2}{2 \times 3 = 6(2) = 3} = \dfrac{2}{3}$

17. $\dfrac{1}{3} \div \dfrac{7}{8} = \dfrac{1 \times 8 = 8}{3 \times 7 = 21} = \dfrac{8}{21}$

18. $\dfrac{1}{5} \div \dfrac{1}{2} = \dfrac{1 \times 2 = 2}{5 \times 1 = 5} = \dfrac{2}{5}$

19. $\dfrac{4}{8} \div \dfrac{2}{3} = \dfrac{4 \times 3 = 12(4) = 3}{8 \times 2 = 16(4) = 4} = \dfrac{3}{4}$

20. $\dfrac{1}{3} \div \dfrac{2}{3} = \dfrac{1 \times 3 = 3(3) = 1}{3 \times 2 = 6(3) = 2} = \dfrac{1}{2}$

21. 0.5

22. 0.33 = 0.3

23. 0.75 = 0.8

24. 0.66 = 0.7

25. 0.125 = 0.1

26.
```
      6.45 (2 decimal points)
    ×1.36 (2 decimal points)
     3870
    19350
    64500
    87720
   8.7720 (4 decimal points from right to left)
```

27.
```
      3.14 (2 decimal points)
    ×2.20 (2 decimal points)
      000
     6280
    62800
    69080
   6.9080 (4 decimal points from right to left)
```

28.   16.286 (3 decimal points)
         ×0.125 (3 decimal points)
            81430
           325720
          1628600
          2035750
          2.035750 (6 decimal points from right to left)

29.   1.2 (1 decimal point)
        ×0.5 (1 decimal point)
          60
         000
         060
        0.60 (2 decimal points from right to left)

30.   7.68 (2 decimal points)
        ×0.05 (2 decimal points)
           3840
           0000
          00000
          03840
         0.3840 (4 decimal points from right to left)

31. 0.5)‾1.25‾

(Move decimal points one place to the right)

Answer: 2.5 = 2.5

$$
\begin{array}{r}
2.5 \\
5)\overline{12.5} \\
\underline{10} \\
2\,5 \\
\underline{2\,5} \\
0
\end{array}
$$

32. 0.20)‾40.80‾

(Move decimal points two places to the right)

Answer: 204. = 204

(Problem continues on next page)

○ **Chapter 1** continued

$$\begin{array}{r} 204 \\ 20\overline{)4080} \\ \underline{40} \\ 080 \\ \underline{80} \\ 0 \end{array}$$

33. $0.125\overline{)0.25}$

    (Move decimal points three places to the right)

    Answer: 2. = 2

$$\begin{array}{r} 2 \\ 125\overline{)250} \\ \underline{250} \\ 0 \end{array}$$

34. $0.75\overline{)0.125}$

    (Move decimal points two places to the right)

    Answer: 0.166 = 0.2

$$\begin{array}{r} .166 \\ 75\overline{)12.500} \\ \underline{7\,5} \\ 5\,00 \\ \underline{4\,50} \\ 50 \end{array}$$

35. $0.5\overline{)7.30}$

    (Move decimal point one place to the left)

    Answer: 14.6 = 14.6

$$\begin{array}{r} 14.6 \\ 5\overline{)73.0} \\ \underline{5} \\ 23 \\ \underline{20} \\ 3\,0 \\ \underline{3\,0} \\ 0 \end{array}$$

CHAPTER 2

1. kilogram = kg
2. gram = g
3. milligram = mg
4. microgram = mcg
5. liter = L
6. milliliter = mL
7. cubic centimeter = cc

1. pound = lb
2. ounce = oz
3. dram = dr
4. grain = gr
5. gallon = gal
6. quart = qt
7. pint = pt
8. fluid ounce = foz
9. fluid dram = fdr
10. minim = M

1. tablespoon = tbsp
2. teaspoon = tsp
3. drop = gtt

1. 1 kg = 2.2 lb
2. 1 kg = 1000 g
3. 1 g = 1000 mg
4. 1 mg = 1000 mcg
5. 1 g = 15 gr
6. 1 gr = 60 mg
7. 1000 mg = 1 g
8. 1000 mL = 1 L = 1 qt
9. 500 mL = 1 pt
10. 240 mL = 8 oz
11. 30 mL = 1 oz = 2 tbsp
12. 15 mL = $\frac{1}{2}$ oz = 3 tsp
13. 5 mL = 1 tsp
14. 1 mL = 15 M = 15 gtt
15. 1 mL = 1 cc

CHAPTER 3

Exercise 1

1. Problem: 4 mg = How many g?
   Given quantity   = 4 mg
   Wanted quantity   = g
   Conversion factor = 1 g = 1000 mg

$$\frac{4 \text{ mg}}{} \bigg| \frac{1 \text{ (g)}}{1000 \text{ mg}} \bigg| \frac{4 \times 1}{1000} \bigg| \frac{4}{1000} = 0.004 \text{ g}$$

2. Problem: 5000 g = How many kg?
   Given quantity   = 5000 g
   Wanted quantity   = kg
   Conversion factor = 1 kg = 1000 g

$$\frac{5000 \text{ gm}}{} \bigg| \frac{1 \text{ (kg)}}{1000 \text{ gm}} \bigg| \frac{5 \times 1}{1} \bigg| \frac{5}{1} = 5 \text{ kg}$$

3. Problem: 0.3 L = How many cc?
   Given quantity   = 0.3 L
   Wanted quantity   = cc
   Conversion factor = 1 L = 1000 cc

$$\frac{0.3 \text{ L}}{} \bigg| \frac{1000 \text{ (cc)}}{1 \text{ L}} \bigg| \frac{0.3 \times 1000}{1} \bigg| \frac{300}{1} = 300 \text{ cc}$$

4. Problem: 10 cc = How many mL?
   Given quantity   = 10 cc
   Wanted quantity   = mL
   Conversion factor = 1 cc = 1 mL

$$\frac{10 \text{ cc}}{} \bigg| \frac{1 \text{ (mL)}}{1 \text{ cc}} \bigg| \frac{10 \times 1}{1} \bigg| \frac{10}{1} = 10 \text{ mL}$$

5. Problem: 120 lb = How many kg?
   Given quantity   = 120 lb
   Wanted quantity   = kg
   Conversion factor = 2.2 lb = 1 kg

$$\frac{120 \text{ lb}}{} \bigg| \frac{1 \text{ (kg)}}{2.2 \text{ lb}} \bigg| \frac{120 \times 1}{2.2} \bigg| \frac{120}{2.2} = 54.5 \text{ kg}$$

6. Problem: 5 gr = How many mg?
   Given quantity   = 5 gr
   Wanted quantity   = mg
   Conversion factor = 1 gr = 60 mg

$$\frac{5 \text{ gr} \mid 60 \text{ (mg)}}{\mid 1 \text{ gr}} \quad \frac{5 \times 60}{1} \quad \frac{300}{1} = 300 \text{ mg}$$

7. Problem: 2 g = How many gr?
   Given quantity   = 2 g
   Wanted quantity   = gr
   Conversion factor = 1 g = 15 gr

$$\frac{2 \text{ g} \mid 15 \text{ (gr)}}{\mid 1 \text{ g}} \quad \frac{2 \times 15}{1} \quad \frac{30}{1} = 30 \text{ gr}$$

8. Problem: 5 fdr = How many mL?
   Given quantity   = 5 fdr
   Wanted quantity   = mL
   Conversion factor = 1 fdr = 5 mL

$$\frac{5 \text{ fdr} \mid 5 \text{ (mL)}}{\mid 1 \text{ fdr}} \quad \frac{5 \times 5}{1} \quad \frac{25}{1} = 25 \text{ mL}$$

9. Problem: 8 fdr = How many foz?
   Given quantity   = 8 fdr
   Wanted quantity   = foz
   Conversion factor = 1 fdr = 5 mL
   Conversion factor = 1 foz = 30 mL

$$\frac{8 \text{ fdr} \mid 5 \text{ mL} \mid 1 \text{ (foz)}}{\mid 1 \text{ fdr} \mid 30 \text{ mL}} \quad \frac{8 \times 5 \times 1}{1 \times 30} \quad \frac{40}{30} = 1.3 \text{ foz}$$

10. Problem: 10 M = How many fdr?
    Given quantity   = M
    Wanted quantity   = fdr
    Conversion factor = 1 mL = 15 M
    Conversion factor = 1 fdr = 5 mL

$$\frac{10 \text{ M} \mid 1 \text{ mL} \mid 1 \text{ (fdr)}}{\mid 15 \text{ M} \mid 5 \text{ mL}} \quad \frac{10 \times 1 \times 1}{15 \times 5} \quad \frac{10}{75} = 0.13 \text{ fdr}$$

◯ **Chapter 3** continued

11. Problem: 35 kg = How many lb?
    Given quantity   = 35 kg
    Wanted quantity   = lb
    Conversion factor = 1 kg = 2.2 lb

$$\frac{35 \ \text{kg} \ | \ 2.2 \ \textcircled{lb}}{| \ 1 \ \text{kg} \ |} \ \frac{| \ 35 \times 2.2}{| \ 1} \ \frac{| \ 77}{| \ 1} = 77 \ \text{lb}$$

12. Problem: 10 mL = How many tsp?
    Given quantity   = 10 mL
    Wanted quantity   = tsp
    Conversion factor = 1 tsp = 5 mL

$$\frac{10 \ \text{mL} \ | \ 1 \ \textcircled{tsp}}{| \ 5 \ \text{mL}} \ \frac{| \ 10 \times 1}{| \ 5} \ \frac{| \ 10}{| \ 5} = 2 \ \text{tsp}$$

13. Problem: 30 mL = How many tbsp?
    Given quantity   = 30 mL
    Wanted quantity   = tbsp
    Conversion factor = 1 tbsp = 15 mL

$$\frac{30 \ \text{mL} \ | \ 1 \ \textcircled{tbsp}}{| \ 15 \ \text{mL}} \ \frac{| \ 30 \times 1}{| \ 15} \ \frac{| \ 30}{| \ 15} = 2 \ \text{tbsp}$$

14. Problem: 0.25 g = How many mg?
    Given quantity   = 0.25 g
    Wanted quantity   = mg
    Conversion factor = 1 g = 1000 mg

$$\frac{0.25 \ \text{g} \ | \ 1000 \ \textcircled{mg}}{| \ 1 \ \text{g}} \ \frac{| \ 0.25 \times 1000}{| \ 1} \ \frac{| \ 250}{| \ 1} = 250 \ \text{mg}$$

15. Problem: 350 mcg = How many mg?
    Given quantity   = 350 mcg
    Wanted quantity   = mg
    Conversion factor = 1 mg = 1000 mcg

$$\frac{350 \ \text{mcg} \ | \ 1 \ \textcircled{mg}}{| \ 1000 \ \text{mcg}} \ \frac{| \ 350}{| \ 1000} = 0.35 \ \text{mg}$$

16. Problem: 0.75 L = How many mL?
Given quantity   = 0.75 L
Wanted quantity   = mL
Conversion factor = 1 L = 1000 mL

$$\frac{0.75 \; \cancel{L} \; | \; 1000 \; (mL)}{| \; 1 \; \cancel{L}} \; \frac{0.75 \times 1000}{1} \; \frac{750}{1} = 750 \text{ mL}$$

17. Problem: 3 hr = How many minutes?
Given quantity   = 3 hr
Wanted quantity   = minutes
Conversion factor = 1 hr = 60 min

$$\frac{3 \; \cancel{hr} \; | \; 60 \; (min)}{| \; 1 \; \cancel{hr}} \; \frac{3 \times 60}{1} \; \frac{180}{1} = 180 \text{ min}$$

18. Problem: 35 mL = How many M?
Given quantity   = 3.5 mL
Wanted quantity   = M
Conversion factor = 1 mL = 15 M

$$\frac{3.5 \; \cancel{mL} \; | \; 15 \; (M)}{| \; 1 \; \cancel{mL}} \; \frac{3.5 \times 15}{1} \; \frac{52.5}{1} = 52.5 \text{ M}$$

19. Problem: 500 mcg = How many mg?
Given quantity   = 500 mcg
Wanted quantity   = mg
Conversion factor = 1 mg = 1000 mcg

$$\frac{500 \; \cancel{mcg} \; | \; 1 \; (mg)}{| \; 1000 \; \cancel{mcg}} \; \frac{500 \times 1}{1000} \; \frac{500}{1000} = 0.5 \text{ mg}$$

20. Problem: 225 M = How many tsp?
Given quantity   = 225 M
Wanted quantity   = tsp
Conversion factor = 1 mL = 15 M
Conversion factor = 1 tsp = 5 mL

$$\frac{225 \; \cancel{M} \; | \; 1 \; \cancel{mL} \; | \; 1 \; (tsp)}{| \; 15 \; \cancel{M} \; | \; 5 \; \cancel{mL}} \; \frac{225 \times 1 \times 1}{15 \times 5} \; \frac{225}{75} = 3 \text{ tsp}$$

◯ **Chapter 3** continued

Practice Problems

1. Problem: $\frac{3}{4}$ mL = How many M?

   Given quantity   = $\frac{3}{4}$ mL
   Wanted quantity   = M
   Conversion factor = 1 mL = 15 M

$$\frac{\frac{3}{4}\ \text{mL} \left| 15\ \text{\textcircled{M}} \right| \frac{3}{4} \times 15 \left| \frac{3}{4} \times \frac{15}{1} \right| \frac{45}{4}}{1\ \text{mL} \quad 1 \quad 1 \quad 1} = 11.25\ \text{M}$$

2. Problem: gtt XV = How many M?
   Given quantity   = 15 gtt
   Wanted quantity   = M
   Conversion factor = 1 gtt = 1 M

$$\frac{15\ \text{gtt} \left| 1\ \text{\textcircled{M}} \right| 15}{1\ \text{gtt}} = 15\ \text{M}$$

3. Problem: $\frac{5}{6}$ gr = How many mg?

   Given quantity   = $\frac{5}{6}$ gr
   Wanted quantity   = mg
   Conversion factor = 1 gr = 60 mg

$$\frac{\frac{5}{6}\ \text{gr} \left| 60\ \text{\textcircled{mg}} \right| \frac{5}{6} \times 60 \left| \frac{5}{6} \times \frac{60}{1} \right| \frac{300}{6} \left| 50 \right.}{1\ \text{gr} \quad 1 \quad 1 \quad 1 \quad 1} = 50\ \text{mg}$$

4. Problem: How many mL in 3 oz?
   Given quantity   = 3 oz
   Wanted quantity   = mL
   Conversion factor = 1 oz = 30 mL

$$\frac{3\ \text{oz} \left| 30\ \text{\textcircled{mL}} \right| 3 \times 30 \left| 90 \right.}{1\ \text{oz} \quad 1 \quad 1} = 90\ \text{mL}$$

5. Problem: 0.5 mg = How many mcg?
   Given quantity   = 0.5 mg

Wanted quantity = mcg
Conversion factor = 1 mg = 1000 mcg

$$\frac{0.5 \text{ mg} \mid 1000 \text{ (mcg)}}{\mid 1 \text{ mg}} \quad \frac{0.5 \times 1000 \mid 500}{1 \mid 1} = 500 \text{ mcg}$$

6. Problem: 35 gtt = How many mL?
   Given quantity   = 35 gtt
   Wanted quantity   = mL
   Conversion factor = 1 gtt = 1 M
   Conversion factor = 15 M = 1 mL

$$\frac{35 \text{ gtt} \mid 1 \text{ M} \mid 1 \text{ (mL)}}{\mid 1 \text{ gtt} \mid 15 \text{ M}} \quad \frac{35 \times 1 \times 1 \mid 35}{1 \times 15 \mid 15} = 2.3 \text{ mL}$$

7. Problem: How many cc in 3 qt?
   Given quantity   = 3 qt
   Wanted quantity   = cc
   Conversion factor = 1 qt = 1000 mL
   Conversion factor = 1 cc = 1 mL

$$\frac{3 \text{ qt} \mid 1000 \text{ mL} \mid 1 \text{ (cc)}}{\mid 1 \text{ qt} \mid 1 \text{ mL}} \quad \frac{3 \times 1000 \times 1 \mid 3000}{1 \mid 1} = 3000 \text{ cc}$$

8. Problem: 4 gal = How many qt?
   Given quantity   = 4 gal
   Wanted quantity   = qt
   Conversion factor = 1 gal = 4 qt

$$\frac{4 \text{ gal} \mid 4 \text{ (qt)}}{\mid 1 \text{ gal}} \quad \frac{4 \times 4 \mid 16}{1 \mid 1} = 16 \text{ qt}$$

9. Problem: 1.5 cup = How many cc?
   Given quantity   = 1.5 cup
   Wanted quantity   = cc
   Conversion factor = 1 cup = 180 cc

$$\frac{1.5 \text{ cup} \mid 180 \text{ (cc)}}{\mid 1 \text{ cup}} \quad \frac{1.5 \times 180 \mid 270}{1 \mid 1} = 270 \text{ cc}$$

10. Problem: 24 oz = How many glasses?
    Given quantity   = 24 oz

(Problem continues on next page)

Wanted quantity = glasses
Conversion factor = 1 glass = 8 oz

$$\frac{24 \text{ oz}}{} \left| \frac{1 \text{ (glass)}}{8 \text{ oz}} \right. = \frac{24 \times 1}{8} = \frac{24}{8} = 3 \text{ glasses}$$

CHAPTER 4

Medication Order #1

Give gr 10 aspirin to Mrs. C. Clark orally every 4 hours as needed for fever.

1. Right patient   Mrs. C. Clark
2. Right drug   Aspirin/for fever
3. Right dosage   gr 10
4. Right route   orally (PO)
5. Right time   every 4 hr as needed (prn)

Medication Order #2

Administer PO to Mr. S. Smith, Advil (ibuprofen) 400 mg every 6 hours for arthritis.

1. Right patient   Mr. S. Smith
2. Right drug   Advil (ibuprofen) for arthritis
3. Right dosage   400 mg
4. Right route   PO (orally)
5. Right time   every 6 hr

Medication Order #3

Tylenol (acetaminophen) gr 10 PO every 4 hours for Mr. J. Jones prn for headache.

1. Right patient   Mr. J. Jones
2. Right drug   Tylenol (acetaminophen)/for headache
3. Right dosage   gr 10
4. Right route   PO (orally)
5. Right time   every 4 hr prn

Practice Problems

1. Sequential method:

$$\frac{0.25 \text{ g}}{} \left| \frac{1000 \text{ mg}}{1 \text{ g}} \right| \frac{\text{(capsule)}}{250 \text{ mg}} = \frac{0.25 \times 100}{1 \times 25} = \frac{25}{25} = 1 \text{ capsule}$$

Random method:

$$\frac{0.25 \text{ g} \, \boxed{\text{capsule}} \, | 1000 \text{ mg} | 0.25 \times 100}{| 250 \text{ mg} | \quad 1 \text{ g} \quad | \quad 25 \times 1} \left| \frac{25}{25} \right. = 1 \text{ capsule}$$

2. Sequential method:

$$\frac{\frac{1}{2} \text{ gr} \, | 60 \text{ mg} \, \boxed{\text{tablet}} \, | \frac{1}{2} \times \frac{60}{1} \left| \frac{60}{2} \right.}{| 15 \text{ mg} | \, 1 \text{ gr} \, | 15 \times 1 \, | 15} \left| \frac{30}{15} \right. = 2 \text{ tablets}$$

Random method:

$$\frac{\frac{1}{2} \text{ gr} \, \boxed{\text{tablet}} \, | 60 \text{ mg} | \frac{1}{2} \times \frac{60}{1} \left| \frac{60}{2} \right.}{| 15 \text{ mg} | \, 1 \text{ gr} \, | 15 \times 1 \, | 15} \left| \frac{30}{15} \right. = 2 \text{ tablets}$$

3. Sequential method:

$$\frac{0.5 \text{ g} \, | 1000 \text{ mg} \, \boxed{\text{tablet}} \, | 0.5 \times 10}{| \quad 1 \text{ g} \quad | 500 \text{ mg} | \, 1 \times 5} \left| \frac{5}{5} \right. = 1 \text{ tablet}$$

Random method:

$$\frac{0.5 \text{ g} \, \boxed{\text{tablet}} \, | 1000 \text{ mg} | 0.5 \times 10}{| 500 \text{ mg} | \quad 1 \text{ g} \quad | \, 5 \times 1} \left| \frac{5}{5} \right. = 1 \text{ tablet}$$

4. Sequential method:

$$\frac{0.03 \text{ g} \, | 1000 \text{ mg} \, \boxed{\text{capsules}} \, | 0.03 \times 100}{| \quad 1 \text{ g} \quad | \, 30 \text{ mg} \, | \quad 1 \times 3} \left| \frac{3}{3} \right. = 1 \text{ capsule}$$

Random method:

$$\frac{0.03 \text{ g} \, \boxed{\text{capsules}} \, | 1000 \text{ mg} | 0.03 \times 100}{| \, 30 \text{ mg} \, | \quad 1 \text{ g} \quad | \, 3 \times 1} \left| \frac{3}{3} \right. = 1 \text{ capsule}$$

○ **Chapter 4** continued

5. Sequential method:

$$\frac{\frac{1}{2} \text{ gr} \left| 60 \text{ mg} \right| \text{spansules}}{1 \text{ gr} \quad \left| 30 \text{ mg} \right|} \frac{\frac{1}{2} \times \frac{60}{1} \left| \frac{60}{2} \right| 30}{1 \times 30 \left| 30 \right| 30} = 1 \text{ spansule}$$

Random method:

$$\frac{\frac{1}{2} \text{ gr} \left| \text{spansules} \right| 60 \text{ mg}}{30 \text{ mg} \quad \left| 1 \text{ gr} \right|} \frac{\frac{1}{2} \times \frac{60}{1} \left| \frac{60}{2} \right| 30}{30 \times 1 \left| 30 \right| 30} = 1 \text{ spansule}$$

Practice Problems With Drug Labels

1. Sequential method:

$$\frac{10 \text{ mg} \left| \text{tablet} \right| 10}{\left| 10 \text{ mg} \right| 10} = 1 \text{ tablet}$$

2. Random method:

$$\frac{500 \text{ mcg} \left| \text{tablet} \right| \quad 1 \text{ mg} \quad \left| 5 \times 1 \right| 5}{\left| 1 \text{ mg} \right| 1000 \text{ mcg} \left| 1 \times 10 \right| 10} = \frac{1}{2} \text{ tablet}$$

3. Sequential method:

$$\frac{375 \text{ mg} \left| \text{tablet} \right| 375}{\left| 250 \text{ mg} \right| 250} = 1\frac{1}{2} \text{ tablets}$$

4. Random method:

$$\frac{2.5 \text{ mg} \left| \text{tablet} \right| \quad \left| 1000 \text{ mcg} \right| 2.5 \times 10 \left| 25 \right.}{\left| 2500 \text{ mcg} \right| \quad 1 \text{ mg} \quad \left| 25 \times 1 \right| 25} = 1 \text{ tablet}$$

5. Sequential method:

$$\frac{250 \text{ mg} \left| \text{capsule} \right| 25}{\left| 250 \text{ mg} \right| 25} = 1 \text{ capsule}$$

Practice Problems With Liquid Medication

1. Random method:

$$\frac{\frac{1}{2}\ \text{gr}}{} \left| \frac{5\ \textcircled{mL}}{20\ \text{mg}} \right| \frac{60\ \text{mg}}{1\ \text{gr}} \left| \frac{\frac{1}{2} \times \frac{5}{1} \times \frac{6}{1}}{2 \times 1} \right| \frac{15}{2} = 7.5\ \text{mL}$$

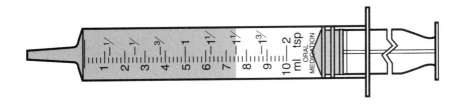

2. Sequential method:

$$\frac{0.15\ \text{g}}{} \left| \frac{1000\ \text{mg}}{1\ \text{g}} \right| \frac{\text{mL}}{15\ \text{mg}} \left| \frac{1}{5\ \text{mL}} \right| \frac{\textcircled{tsp}}{} \left| \frac{0.15 \times 1000}{15 \times 5} \right| \frac{150}{75} = 2\ \text{tsp}$$

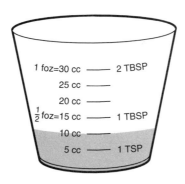

3. Sequential method:

$$\frac{3\ \text{mg}}{} \left| \frac{\textcircled{mL}}{1\ \text{mg}} \right| \frac{3}{1} = 3\ \text{mL}$$

(Problem continues on next page)

○ **Chapter 4** continued

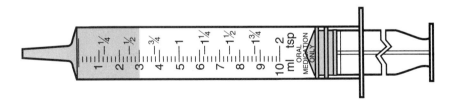

4. Sequential method:

$$\frac{20\ \cancel{g}}{}\ \bigg|\frac{15\ \cancel{mL}}{10\ \cancel{g}}\ \bigg|\frac{1\ \textcircled{oz}}{30\ \cancel{mL}}\ \bigg|\frac{2 \times 15 \times 1}{1 \times 30}\ \bigg|\frac{30}{30} = 1\ oz$$

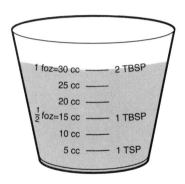

Practice Problems With Parenteral Medications

1. Random method:

$$\frac{300\ \cancel{mcg}}{}\ \bigg|\frac{\textcircled{mL}}{0.1\ \cancel{mg}}\ \bigg|\frac{1\ \cancel{mg}}{1000\ \cancel{mcg}}\ \bigg|\frac{3 \times 1}{0.1 \times 10}\ \bigg|\frac{3}{1} = 3\ mL$$

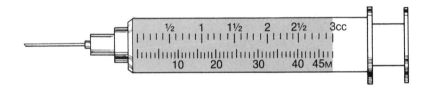

2. Sequential method:

$$\frac{3\ \text{mg}\ \boxed{\text{mL}}\ |3}{|2\ \text{mg}|2} = 1.5\ \text{mL}$$

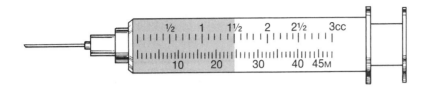

3. Sequential method:

$$\frac{35\ \text{mg}\ |\ \boxed{\text{mL}}\ |35}{|10\ \text{mg}|10} = 3.5\ \text{mL}$$

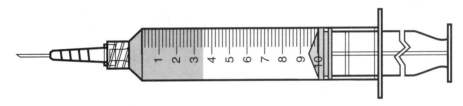

4. Sequential method:

$$\frac{10\ \text{units}}{} \qquad = 10\ \text{units}$$

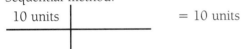

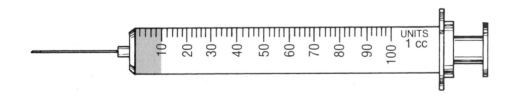

5. Sequential method:

$$\frac{8{,}000\ \text{units}|\ \boxed{\text{mL}}\ |8}{|10{,}000\ \text{units}|10} = 0.8\ \text{mL}$$

(Problem continues on next page)

◯ **Chapter 4** continued

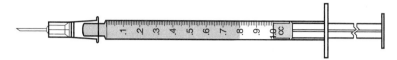

Practice Problems

1. Random method:

$$\frac{0.2 \text{ g}}{} \left| \frac{\text{mL}}{100 \text{ mg}} \right| \frac{1000 \text{ mg}}{1 \text{ g}} \right| \frac{0.2 \times 10}{1 \times 1} \right| \frac{2}{1} = 2 \text{ mL}$$

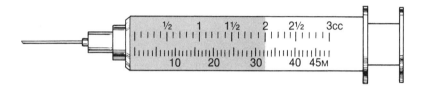

2. Sequential method:

$$\frac{50 \text{ mg}}{} \left| \frac{\text{tablet}}{25 \text{ mg}} \right| \frac{50}{25} = 2 \text{ tablets}$$

3. Random method:

$$\frac{1 \text{ g}}{} \left| \frac{\text{tablet}}{500 \text{ mg}} \right| \frac{1000 \text{ mg}}{1 \text{ g}} \right| \frac{1 \times 10}{5 \times 1} \right| \frac{10}{5} = 2 \text{ tablets}$$

4. Random method:

$$\frac{50 \text{ mg}}{} \left| \frac{\text{tablet}}{25 \text{ mg}} \right| \frac{50}{25} = 2 \text{ tablets}$$

5. Sequential method:

$$\frac{56 \text{ units}}{} \left| = 56 \text{ units} \right.$$

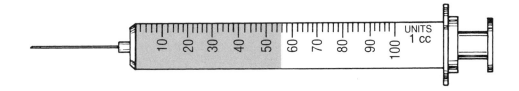

6. Sequential method:

$$\frac{7500 \text{ units}}{} \left| \frac{\text{mL}}{10,000 \text{ units}} \right| \frac{75}{100} = 0.75 \text{ mL}$$

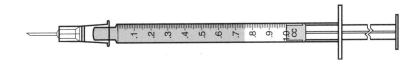

7. Sequential method:

$$\frac{500 \text{ mg}}{} \left| \frac{5 \text{ mL}}{125 \text{ mg}} \right| \frac{500 \times 5}{125} \left| \frac{2500}{125} \right. = 20 \text{ mL}$$

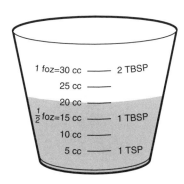

8. Sequential method:

$$\frac{5 \text{ mg}}{} \left| \frac{\text{tablet}}{2.5 \text{ mg}} \right| \frac{5}{2.5} = 2 \text{ tablets}$$

⊖ **Chapter 4** continued

9. Sequential method:

$$\frac{10 \ \text{mg} \ \boxed{\text{capsule}} \ 10}{10 \ \text{mg} \ | 10} = 1 \ \text{capsule}$$

10. Sequential method:

$$\frac{50 \ \text{mg} \ \boxed{\text{mL}} \ 5}{100 \ \text{mg} \ | 10} = 0.5 \ \text{mL}$$

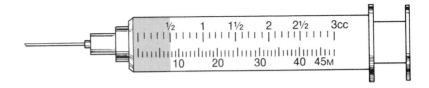

CHAPTER 5

Practice Problems Involving Weight

1. Sequential method:

$$\frac{1 \ \text{mg} \ \boxed{\text{mL}} \ 1 \ \text{kg} \ 45 \ \text{lb}}{\text{kg} \ | 10 \ \text{mg} | 2.2 \ \text{lb}} \ \frac{1 \times 1 \times 45}{10 \times 2.2} \ \frac{45}{22} = 2.04 \ \text{or} \ 2 \ \text{mL}$$

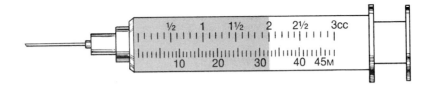

2. Sequential method:

$$\frac{0.01 \ \text{mg} \ \boxed{\text{mL}} \ 1 \ \text{kg} \ 20 \ \text{lb}}{\text{kg} \ | 0.1 \ \text{mg} | 2.2 \ \text{lb}} \ \frac{0.01 \times 1 \times 20}{0.1 \times 2.2} \ \frac{0.2}{0.22} = 0.9 \ \text{mL}$$

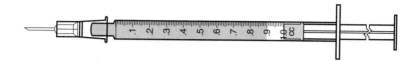

3. Sequential method:

$$\frac{0.5 \text{ mg}}{\text{kg}} \left|\frac{\text{mL}}{25 \text{ mg}}\right| \frac{1 \text{ kg}}{2.2 \text{ lb}} \left|\frac{45 \text{ lb}}{}\right| \frac{0.5 \times 1 \times 45}{25 \times 2.2} \left|\frac{22.5}{55}\right| = 0.4 \text{ mL}$$

4. Random method:

$$\frac{500 \text{ mcg}}{\text{kg}} \left|\frac{\text{mL}}{8 \text{ mg}}\right| \frac{1 \text{ mg}}{1000 \text{ mcg}} \left|\frac{1 \text{ kg}}{2.2 \text{ lb}}\right| \frac{75 \text{ lb}}{} \left|\frac{5 \times 1 \times 1 \times 75}{8 \times 10 \times 2.2}\right| \frac{375}{176} = \text{mL}$$

$$\frac{375}{176} = 2.13 \text{ or } 2 \text{ mL}$$

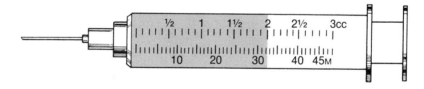

5. Random method:

$$\frac{10 \text{ mg}}{\text{kg}} \left|\frac{1 \text{ kg}}{2.2 \text{ lb}}\right| \frac{70 \text{ lb}}{} \left|\frac{5 \text{ mL}}{300 \text{ mg}}\right| \frac{10 \times 1 \times 7 \times 5}{2.2 \times 30} \left|\frac{350}{66}\right| = 5.3 \text{ or } 5 \text{ mL}$$

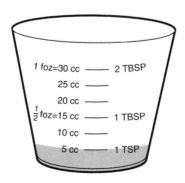

○ **Chapter 5** continued

Practice Problems Involving Reconstitution

1. Random method:

$$\frac{500 \text{ mg} \; | \; 50 \; (\text{mL}) \; | \quad 1 \text{ g} \quad |}{ \quad | \quad 1 \text{ g} \; | \; 1000 \text{ mg} \; |} \; \frac{5 \times 5}{1} \Big| \frac{25}{1} = 25 \text{ mL}$$

2. Sequential method:

$$\frac{250 \text{ mg} \; | \; 10 \; (\text{mL}) }{ \quad | \; 500 \text{ mg}} \Big| \frac{25 \times 1}{5} \Big| \frac{25}{5} = 5 \text{ mL}$$

3. Random method:

$$\frac{50 \text{ mg} \; | \; 4 \; (\text{mL}) \; | \quad 1 \text{ g} \quad | \; 40 \text{ kg}}{\text{kg} \quad | \; 1.5 \text{ g} \; | \; 1000 \text{ mg} |} \; \frac{5 \times 4 \times 1 \times 4}{1.5 \times 10} \Big| \frac{80}{15} = 5.33 \text{ or } 5 \text{ mL}$$

Random method using yield:

$$\frac{50 \text{ mg} \; | \; 1 \; (\text{mL}) \; | \; 40 \text{ kg}}{\text{kg} \quad | \; 375 \text{ mg} |} \; \frac{50 \times 1 \times 40}{375} \Big| \frac{2000}{375} = 5.33 \text{ or } 5 \text{ mL}$$

4. Random method:

$$\frac{750 \text{ mg} \; | \; 20 \; (\text{mL}) \; | \quad 1 \text{ g} \quad |}{\quad | \; 1 \text{ g} \; | \; 1000 \text{ mg} |} \; \frac{75 \times 2 \times 1}{1 \times 10} \Big| \frac{150}{10} = 15 \text{ mL}$$

5. Sequential method:

$$\frac{30 \text{ mg} \; | \; 5 \; (\text{mL}) \; | \; 1 \text{ kg} \; | \; 65 \text{ lb}}{\text{kg} \quad | \; 500 \text{ mg} | \; 2.2 \text{ lb} |} \; \frac{3 \times 5 \times 1 \times 65}{50 \times 2.2} \Big| \frac{975}{110} = 8.86 \text{ or } 8.9 \text{ mL}$$

Practice Problems Involving
Intravenous Pumps

1. Sequential method:

$$\frac{1800 \text{ units}}{\text{hr}} \left| \frac{250 \text{ mL}}{25,000 \text{ units}} \right| 18 = \frac{18 \text{ mL}}{\text{hr}}$$

2. Random method:

$$\frac{35 \text{ mg}}{\text{hr}} \left| \frac{250 \text{ mL}}{1 \text{ g}} \right| \frac{1 \text{ g}}{1000 \text{ mg}} \left| \frac{35 \times 25}{100} \right| \frac{875}{100} = 8.75 \text{ or } \frac{9 \text{ mL}}{\text{hr}}$$

3. Sequential method:

$$\frac{30 \text{ mL}}{\text{hr}} \left| \frac{25,000 \text{ units}}{250 \text{ mL} 25} \right| \frac{30 \times 2500}{25} \left| \frac{75000}{25} \right| = 3,000 \frac{\text{units}}{\text{hr}}$$

4. Sequential method:

$$\frac{15 \text{ mL}}{\text{hr}} \left| \frac{1 \text{ g}}{250 \text{ mL}} \right| \frac{1000 \text{ mg}}{1 \text{ g}} \left| \frac{15 \times 100}{25} \right| \frac{1500}{25} = 60 \frac{\text{mg}}{\text{hr}}$$

5. Sequential method:

$$\frac{900 \text{ units}}{\text{hr}} \left| \frac{500 \text{ mL}}{25,000 \text{ units}} \right| \frac{90 \times 5}{25} \left| \frac{450}{25} \right| = \frac{18 \text{ mL}}{\text{hr}}$$

Practice Problems Involving Drop Factors

1. Sequential method:

$$\frac{800 \text{ mL}}{8 \text{ hr}} \left| \frac{15 \text{ gtt}}{\text{mL}} \right| \frac{1 \text{ hr}}{60 \text{ min}} \left| \frac{80 \times 15 \times 1}{8 \times 6} \right| \frac{1200}{48} = 25 \frac{\text{gtt}}{\text{min}}$$

○ **Chapter 5** continued

2. Sequential method:

$$\frac{250 \text{ mL}}{} \left| \frac{15 \text{ gtt}}{\text{mL}} \right| \frac{\text{min}}{60 \text{ gtt}} \left| \frac{1 \text{ hr}}{60 \text{ min}} \right. \frac{250 \times 15 \times 1}{60 \times 60} \frac{3750}{3600} = 1.04 \text{ or } 1 \text{ hr}$$

3. Sequential method:

$$\frac{150 \text{ mL}}{60 \text{ min}} \left| \frac{10 \text{ gtt}}{\text{mL}} \right. \frac{150 \times 1}{6} \frac{150}{6} = 25 \frac{\text{gtt}}{\text{min}}$$

4. Sequential method:

$$\frac{1000 \text{ mL}}{} \left| \frac{15 \text{ gtt}}{\text{mL}} \right| \frac{\text{min}}{50 \text{ gtt}} \left| \frac{1 \text{ hr}}{60 \text{ min}} \right. \frac{10 \times 15 \times 1}{5 \times 6} \frac{150}{30} = 5 \text{ hr}$$

5. Sequential method:

$$\frac{500 \text{ mL}}{4 \text{ hr}} \left| \frac{15 \text{ gtt}}{\text{mL}} \right| \frac{1 \text{ hr}}{60 \text{ min}} \left. \frac{50 \times 15 \times 1}{4 \times 6} \frac{750}{24} = 31.25 \text{ or } 31 \frac{\text{gtt}}{\text{min}} \right.$$

Practice Problems Involving Intermittent Infusion

1. Random method:

$$\frac{250 \text{ mg}}{} \left| \frac{10 \text{ mL}}{1 \text{ g}} \right| \frac{1 \text{ g}}{1000 \text{ mg}} \left. \frac{25 \times 1}{10} \frac{25}{10} = 2.5 \text{ mL} \right.$$

Calculate milliliters per hour to set the IV pump.
Random method:

$$\frac{52.5 \text{ mL}}{15 \text{ min}} \left| \frac{60 \text{ min}}{1 \text{ hr}} \right. \frac{52.5 \times 60}{15 \times 1} \frac{3150}{15} = 210 \frac{\text{mL}}{\text{hr}}$$

Calculate drops per minute with a drop factor of 10 gtt/mL.

Sequential method:

$$\frac{52.5 \text{ mL}}{15 \text{ min}} \Bigg| \frac{10 \text{ gtt}}{\text{mL}} \Bigg| \frac{52.5 \times 10}{15} \Bigg| \frac{525}{15} = 35 \frac{\text{gtt}}{\text{min}}$$

2. Random method:

$$\frac{0.3 \text{ g}}{} \Bigg| \frac{4 \text{ mL}}{600 \text{ mg}} \Bigg| \frac{1000 \text{ mg}}{1 \text{ g}} \Bigg| \frac{0.3 \times 4 \times 10}{6 \times 1} \Bigg| \frac{12}{6} = 2 \text{ mL}$$

Calculate milliliter per hour to set the IV pump.
Random method:

$$\frac{52 \text{ mL}}{15 \text{ min}} \Bigg| \frac{60 \text{ min}}{1 \text{ hr}} \Bigg| \frac{52 \times 60}{15 \times 1} \Bigg| \frac{3120}{15} = 208 \frac{\text{mL}}{\text{hr}}$$

Calculate drops per minute with a drop factor of 15 gtt/mL.
Sequential method:

$$\frac{52 \text{ mL}}{15 \text{ min}} \Bigg| \frac{15 \text{ gtt}}{\text{mL}} \Bigg| \frac{52}{} = 52 \frac{\text{gtt}}{\text{min}}$$

3. Sequential method:

$$\frac{3 \text{ g}}{} \Bigg| \frac{40 \text{ mL}}{4 \text{ g}} \Bigg| \frac{3 \times 40}{4} \Bigg| \frac{120}{4} = 30 \text{ mL}$$

Calculate milliliters per hour to set the IV pump.
Sequential method:

$$\frac{130 \text{ mL}}{1 \text{ hr}} \Bigg| \frac{130}{1} = 130 \frac{\text{mL}}{\text{hr}}$$

Calculate drops per minute with a drop factor of 20 gtt/mL.
Sequential method:

$$\frac{130 \text{ mL}}{1 \text{ hr}} \Bigg| \frac{20 \text{ gtt}}{\text{mL}} \Bigg| \frac{1 \text{ hr}}{60 \text{ min}} \Bigg| \frac{130 \times 2}{6} \Bigg| \frac{260}{6} = 43.33 \text{ or } 43 \frac{\text{gtt}}{\text{min}}$$

4. Random method:

$$\frac{1000 \text{ mg}}{} \Bigg| \frac{4 \text{ mL}}{1.5 \text{ g}} \Bigg| \frac{1 \text{ g}}{1000 \text{ mg}} \Bigg| \frac{4 \times 1}{1.5} \Bigg| \frac{4}{1.5} = 2.66 \text{ or } 2.7 \text{ mL}$$

○ **Chapter 5** continued

Calculate milliliters per hour to set the IV pump.
Sequential method:

$$\frac{102.7 \;\text{mL}}{1 \;\text{hr}} \Bigg| \frac{102.7}{1} = 102.7 \text{ or } 103 \; \frac{\text{mL}}{\text{hr}}$$

Calculate drops per minute with a drop factor of 20 gtt/mL.

Sequential method:

$$\frac{102.7 \;\text{mL}}{1 \;\text{hr}} \Bigg| \frac{20 \;\text{gtt}}{\text{mL}} \Bigg| \frac{1 \;\text{hr}}{60 \;\text{min}} \Bigg| \frac{102.7 \times 2}{6} \Bigg| \frac{205.4}{6} = 34.2 \text{ or } 34 \; \frac{\text{gtt}}{\text{min}}$$

5. Sequential method:

$$\frac{50 \;\text{mg}}{} \Bigg| \frac{\text{mL}}{25 \;\text{mg}} \Bigg| \frac{50}{25} = 2 \; \text{mL}$$

Calculate milliliters per hour to set the IV pump.
Random method:

$$\frac{52 \;\text{mL}}{30 \;\text{min}} \Bigg| \frac{60 \;\text{min}}{1 \;\text{hr}} \Bigg| \frac{52 \times 6}{3 \times 1} \Bigg| \frac{312}{3} = 104 \; \frac{\text{mL}}{\text{hr}}$$

Calculate drops per minute with a drop factor of 10 gtt/mL.
Sequential method:

$$\frac{52 \;\text{mL}}{30 \;\text{min}} \Bigg| \frac{10 \;\text{gtt}}{\text{mL}} \Bigg| \frac{52 \times 1}{3} \Bigg| \frac{52}{3} = 17.3 \text{ or } 17 \; \frac{\text{gtt}}{\text{min}}$$

Practice Problems

1. Sequential method:

$$\frac{0.2 \;\text{mg}}{\text{kg}} \Bigg| \frac{2 \;\text{mL}}{5 \;\text{mg}} \Bigg| \frac{1 \;\text{kg}}{2.2 \;\text{lb}} \Bigg| \frac{10 \;\text{lb}}{} \Bigg| \frac{0.2 \times 2 \times 1 \times 10}{5 \times 2.2} \Bigg| \frac{4}{11} = 0.36 \text{ or } 0.4 \; \text{mL}$$

2. Sequential method:

$$\frac{10 \text{ mg}}{\text{kg}} \left| \frac{5 \text{ (mL)}}{160 \text{ mg}} \right| \frac{8 \text{ kg}}{} \frac{1 \times 5 \times 8}{16} \left| \frac{40}{16} \right. = 2.5 \text{ mL}$$

3. Sequential method:

$$\frac{1.25 \text{ g}}{} \left| \frac{10 \text{ (mL)}}{2 \text{ g}} \right| \frac{1.25 \times 10}{2} \left| \frac{12.5}{2} \right. = 6.25 \text{ or } 6.3 \text{ mL}$$

4. Random method:

$$\frac{750 \text{ mg}}{} \left| \frac{4 \text{ (mL)}}{1.5 \text{ g}} \right| \frac{1 \text{ g}}{1000 \text{ mg}} \left| \frac{75 \times 4 \times 1}{1.5 \times 100} \right| \frac{300}{150} = 2 \text{ mL}$$

5. Sequential method:

$$\frac{700 \text{ units}}{\text{(hr)}} \left| \frac{250 \text{ (mL)}}{25,000 \text{ units}} \right| \frac{7}{} = \frac{7 \text{ mL}}{\text{hr}}$$

6. Sequential method:

$$\frac{11 \text{ mL}}{\text{(hr)}} \left| \frac{150 \text{ (mg)}}{250 \text{ mL}} \right| \frac{11 \times 15}{25} \left| \frac{165}{25} \right. = \frac{6.6 \text{ mg}}{\text{hr}}$$

7. Sequential method:

$$\frac{1000 \text{ mL}}{8 \text{ hr}} \left| \frac{20 \text{ (gtt)}}{\text{mL}} \right| \frac{1 \text{ hr}}{60 \text{ (min)}} \left| \frac{1000 \times 2 \times 1}{8 \times 6} \right| \frac{2000}{48} = 41.66 \text{ or } 42 \frac{\text{gtt}}{\text{min}}$$

8. Sequential method:

$$\frac{750 \text{ mL}}{} \left| \frac{15 \text{ gtt}}{\text{mL}} \right| \frac{\text{min}}{18 \text{ gtt}} \left| \frac{1 \text{ (hr)}}{60 \text{ min}} \right| \frac{75 \times 15 \times 1}{18 \times 6} \left| \frac{1125}{108} \right. = 10.41 \text{ or } 10 \text{ hr}$$

◯ **Chapter 5** continued

9. Sequential method:

$$\frac{10\ \text{mg}}{\text{kg}} \left| \frac{10\ \text{mL}}{500\ \text{mg}} \right| \frac{1\ \text{kg}}{2.2\ \text{lb}} \left| 20\ \text{lb} \right| \frac{1 \times 1 \times 20}{5 \times 2.2} \left| \frac{20}{11} \right. = 1.8\ \text{mL}$$

Sequential method:

$$\frac{101.8\ \text{mL}}{1\ \text{hr}} \left| \frac{101.8}{1} \right. = 101.8\ \text{or}\ \frac{102\ \text{mL}}{\text{hr}}$$

Sequential method:

$$\frac{101.8\ \text{mL}}{1\ \text{hr}} \left| \frac{10\ \text{gtt}}{\text{mL}} \right| \frac{1\ \text{hr}}{60\ \text{min}} \left| \frac{101.8 \times 1}{6} \right| \frac{101.8}{6} = 16.96\ \text{or}\ 17\ \frac{\text{gtt}}{\text{min}}$$

10. Sequential method: Calculate mL per hour to set the IV pump.

$$\frac{355\ \text{mg}}{} \left| \frac{10\ \text{mL}}{500\ \text{mg}} \right| \frac{355 \times 1}{50} \left| \frac{355}{50} \right. = 7.1\ \text{or}\ 7\ \text{mL} \qquad \frac{107\ \text{mL}}{1\ \text{hr}} \left| \frac{107}{1} \right. = 107\ \frac{\text{mL}}{\text{hr}}$$

Calculate drops per minute with a drop factor of 20 gtt/mL.
Sequential method:

$$\frac{107\ \text{mL}}{1\ \text{hr}} \left| \frac{20\ \text{gtt}}{\text{mL}} \right| \frac{1\ \text{hr}}{60\ \text{min}} \left| \frac{107 \times 2}{6} \right| \frac{214}{6} = 35.66\ \text{or}\ 36\ \frac{\text{gtt}}{\text{min}}$$

CHAPTER 6

Practice Problems Involving Dosage, Weight, and Time

1. Sequential method:

$$\frac{2\ \text{mg}}{\text{kg/day}} \left| \frac{5\ \text{mL}}{40\ \text{mg}} \right| \frac{20\ \text{kg}}{} \left| \frac{\text{day}}{2\ \text{doses}} \right| \frac{2 \times 5 \times 2}{4 \times 2} \left| \frac{20}{8} \right. = 2.5\ \frac{\text{mL}}{\text{dose}}$$

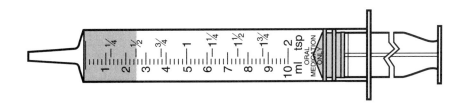

2. Random method:

$$\frac{40 \text{ mg}}{\text{kg/day}} \left| \frac{10 \text{ (mL)}}{1 \text{ g}} \right| \frac{\text{day}}{3 \text{ (doses)}} \left| \frac{1 \text{ kg}}{2.2 \text{ lb}} \right| \frac{30 \text{ lb}}{} \left| \frac{1 \text{ g}}{1000 \text{ mg}} \right| = \frac{\text{mL}}{\text{dose}}$$

$$\frac{4 \times 1 \times 3}{3 \times 2.2} \left| \frac{12}{6.6} \right| = 1.81 \text{ or } 1.8 \frac{\text{mL}}{\text{dose}}$$

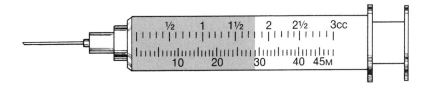

3. Sequential method:

$$\frac{6 \text{ mg}}{\text{kg/day}} \left| \frac{5 \text{ (mL)}}{125 \text{ mg}} \right| \frac{1 \text{ kg}}{2.2 \text{ lb}} \left| \frac{45 \text{ lb}}{} \right| \frac{\text{day}}{2 \text{ (doses)}} = \frac{\text{mL}}{\text{dose}}$$

$$\frac{6 \times 5 \times 1 \times 45}{125 \times 2.2 \times 2} \left| \frac{1350}{550} \right| = 2.45 \text{ or } 2.5 \frac{\text{mL}}{\text{dose}}$$

4. Sequential method:

$$\frac{1.5 \text{ mg}}{\text{kg/day}} \left| \frac{5 \text{ (mL)}}{6.7 \text{ mg}} \right| \frac{20 \text{ kg}}{} \left| \frac{\text{day}}{4 \text{ (doses)}} \right| \frac{1.5 \times 5 \times 20}{6.7 \times 4} = \frac{\text{mL}}{\text{dose}}$$

$$\frac{150}{26.8} = 5.59 \text{ or } 5.6 \frac{\text{mL}}{\text{dose}}$$

○ **Chapter 6** continued

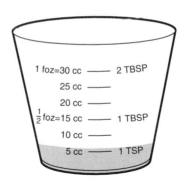

5. Sequential method:

$$\frac{10\ \text{mg}\ |\ 2\ \textcircled{mL}\ |\ 1\ \text{kg}\ |\ 1\ \text{day}\ |\ 50\ \text{lb}\ |\ 1 \times 2 \times 1 \times 1 \times 5|}{\text{kg/day}\ |300\ \text{mg}|2.2\ \text{lb}|3\ \textcircled{doses}|\qquad\ 3 \times 2.2 \times 3} \quad \frac{10}{19.8} = \frac{0.5\ \text{mL}}{\text{dose}}$$

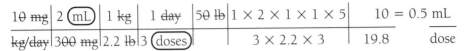

6. Sequential method:

$$\frac{400\ \text{mg}|\ \textcircled{mL}\ |40}{\quad|40\ \text{mg}|\ 4} = 10\ \text{mL}$$

Calculate milliliter to set the IV pump.
Random method:

$$\frac{5\ \text{mcg}\ |60\ \text{min}|\ 1\ \text{kg}\ |200\ \text{lb}|260\ \textcircled{mL}\ |\ 1\ \text{mg}\ }{\text{kg/min}|1\ \textcircled{hr}|2.2\ \text{lb}|\qquad|400\ \text{mg}|1000\ \text{mcg}} = \frac{\text{mL}}{\text{hr}}$$

$$\frac{5 \times 6 \times 2 \times 26 \times 1\ |\ 1560}{2.2 \times 4 \times 10\ \ |\ 88} = \frac{17.7\ \text{or}\ 18\ \text{mL}}{\text{hr}}$$

7. Sequential method:

$$\frac{22\ \text{mL}|\ 50\ \text{mg}\ |\ 1\ \text{hr}\ |1000\ \textcircled{mcg}|2.2\ \text{lb}|}{\text{hr}\ |250\ \text{mL}|60\ \textcircled{min}|\ 1\ \text{mg}\ |1\ \textcircled{kg}|160\ \text{lb}} = \frac{\text{mcg}}{\text{kg/min}}$$

$$\frac{22 \times 5 \times 10 \times 2.2}{25 \times 6 \times 1 \times 16} \Bigg| \frac{2420}{2400} = 1.008 \text{ or } 1 \frac{\text{mcg}}{\text{kg/min}}$$

8. Random method:

$$\frac{5 \text{ mcg}}{\text{kg/min}} \Bigg| \frac{100 \text{ mL}}{100 \text{ mg}} \Bigg| \frac{1 \text{ mg}}{1000 \text{ mcg}} \Bigg| \frac{1 \text{ kg}}{2.2 \text{ lb}} \Bigg| \frac{180 \text{ lb}}{} \Bigg| \frac{60 \text{ min}}{1 \text{ hr}} = \frac{\text{mL}}{\text{hr}}$$

$$\frac{5 \times 1 \times 18 \times 6}{10 \times 2.2} \Bigg| \frac{540}{22} = 24.5 \text{ or } 25 \frac{\text{mL}}{\text{hr}}$$

9. How many micrograms per kilogram per minute is the patient receiving?
Sequential method:

$$\frac{46 \text{ mL}}{\text{hr}} \Bigg| \frac{50 \text{ mg}}{250 \text{ mL}} \Bigg| \frac{1 \text{ hr}}{60 \text{ min}} \Bigg| \frac{1000 \text{ mcg}}{1 \text{ mg}} \Bigg| \frac{2.2 \text{ lb}}{1 \text{ kg}} \Bigg| \frac{}{160 \text{ lb}} = \frac{\text{mcg}}{\text{kg/min}}$$

$$\frac{46 \times 5 \times 10 \times 2.2}{25 \times 6 \times 1 \times 16} \Bigg| \frac{5060}{2400} = 2.1 \text{ or } 2 \frac{\text{mcg}}{\text{kg/min}}$$

10. Sequential method:

$$\frac{500 \text{ mg}}{} \Bigg| \frac{\text{mL}}{50 \text{ mg}} \Bigg| \frac{50}{5} = 10 \text{ mL}$$

Sequential method:

$$\frac{5 \text{ mg}}{\text{kg/30 min}} \Bigg| \frac{60 \text{ mL}}{500 \text{ mg}} \Bigg| \frac{1 \text{ kg}}{2.2 \text{ lb}} \Bigg| \frac{240 \text{ lb}}{} \Bigg| \frac{60 \text{ min}}{1 \text{ hr}} = \frac{\text{mL}}{\text{hr}}$$

$$\frac{5 \times 6 \times 24 \times 6}{3 \times 5 \times 2.2} \Bigg| \frac{4320}{33} = 130.9 \text{ or } 131 \frac{\text{mL}}{\text{hr}}$$

Practice Problems

1. Random method:

$$\frac{8 \text{ mcg}}{\text{kg/min}} \Bigg| \frac{100 \text{ mL}}{100 \text{ mg}} \Bigg| \frac{1 \text{ mg}}{1000 \text{ mcg}} \Bigg| \frac{1 \text{ kg}}{2.2 \text{ lb}} \Bigg| \frac{198 \text{ lb}}{} \Bigg| \frac{60 \text{ min}}{1 \text{ hr}} = \frac{\text{mL}}{\text{hr}}$$

◯ **Chapter 6** continued

$$\frac{8 \times 1 \times 198 \times 6}{100 \times 2.2} \quad \bigg| \quad \frac{9504}{220} \quad = 43.2 \; \frac{\text{mL}}{\text{hr}}$$

2. Sequential method:

$$\frac{40 \; \text{mg}}{\text{kg/day}} \bigg| \frac{5 \; \text{(mL)}}{300 \; \text{mg}} \bigg| \frac{1 \; \text{kg}}{2.2 \; \text{lb}} \bigg| \frac{80 \; \text{lb}}{} \bigg| \frac{\text{day}}{4 \; \text{(doses)}} \quad = \frac{\text{mL}}{\text{dose}}$$

$$\frac{4 \times 5 \times 1 \times 8}{3 \times 2.2 \times 4} \quad \bigg| \quad \frac{160}{26.4} \quad = 6.06 \text{ or } 6 \; \frac{\text{mL}}{\text{dose}}$$

3. Sequential method:

$$\frac{45 \; \text{mL}}{\text{hr}} \bigg| \frac{200 \; \text{mg}}{500 \; \text{mL}} \bigg| \frac{1000 \; \text{(mcg)}}{1 \; \text{mg}} \bigg| \frac{1 \; \text{hr}}{60 \; \text{(min)}} \bigg| \frac{}{60 \; \text{(kg)}} \quad = \frac{\text{mcg}}{\text{kg/min}}$$

$$\frac{45 \times 2 \times 10}{5 \times 6 \times 6} \quad \bigg| \quad \frac{900}{180} \quad = 5 \; \frac{\text{mcg}}{\text{kg/min}}$$

4. Random method:

$$\frac{2 \; \text{mcg}}{\text{kg/min}} \bigg| \frac{500 \; \text{(mL)}}{400 \; \text{mg}} \bigg| \frac{1 \; \text{mg}}{1000 \; \text{mcg}} \bigg| \frac{60 \; \text{min}}{1 \; \text{(hr)}} \bigg| \frac{1 \; \text{kg}}{2.2 \; \text{lb}} \bigg| \frac{176 \; \text{lb}}{} = \frac{\text{mL}}{\text{hr}}$$

$$\frac{2 \times 5 \times 6 \times 1 \times 176}{4 \times 100 \times 2.2} \quad \bigg| \quad \frac{10560}{880} \quad = 12 \; \frac{\text{mL}}{\text{hr}}$$

5. Random method:

$$\frac{5 \; \text{(mcg)}}{\text{kg/(day)}} \bigg| \frac{1 \; \text{kg}}{2.2 \; \text{lb}} \bigg| \frac{130 \; \text{lb}}{} \bigg| \frac{5 \times 1 \times 130}{2.2} \bigg| \frac{650}{2.2} = 295.45 \text{ or } 295 \; \frac{\text{mcg}}{\text{day}}$$

6. Sequential method:

$$\frac{0.5 \; \cancel{mg}}{\cancel{kg}/\cancel{hr}} \left| \frac{\cancel{250} \; \cancel{(mL)}}{250 \; \cancel{mg}} \right| \frac{1 \; \cancel{kg}}{2.2 \; \cancel{lb}} \left| \frac{132 \; \cancel{lb}}{} \right| \frac{0.5 \times 1 \times 132}{2.2} \left| \frac{66}{2.2} \right. = \frac{30 \; mL}{hr}$$

7. Sequential method:

$$\frac{2 \; \cancel{mg}}{\cancel{kg}/\cancel{(day)}} \left| \frac{\cancel{(mL)}}{10 \; \cancel{mg}} \right| \frac{40 \; \cancel{kg}}{} \left| \frac{2 \times 4}{1} \right| \frac{8}{1} = \frac{8 \; mL}{day}$$

8. Sequential method:

$$\frac{15 \; \cancel{mL}}{\cancel{hr}} \left| \frac{200 \; \cancel{mg}}{1000 \; \cancel{mL}} \right| \frac{1 \; \cancel{hr}}{60 \; \cancel{(min)}} \left| \frac{1000 \; \cancel{(mcg)}}{1 \; \cancel{mg}} \right| \frac{}{100 \; \cancel{(kg)}} \left| \frac{15 \times 2}{60} \right| \frac{30}{60} = \frac{0.5 \; mcg}{kg/min}$$

9. Sequential method:

$$\frac{10 \; \cancel{mL}}{\cancel{dose}} \left| \frac{300 \; \cancel{(mg)}}{5 \; \cancel{mL}} \right| \frac{4 \; \cancel{doses}}{\cancel{(day)}} \left| \frac{2.2 \; \cancel{lb}}{1 \; \cancel{(kg)}} \right| \frac{}{65 \; \cancel{lb}} = \frac{mg}{kg/day}$$

$$\frac{10 \times 300 \times 4 \times 2.2}{5 \times 1 \times 65} \left| \frac{26400}{325} \right. = 81.23 \; or \; \frac{81 \; mg}{kg/day}$$

10. Sequential method:

$$\frac{25 \; \cancel{mL}}{\cancel{(hr)}} \left| \frac{\cancel{250} \; \cancel{(mg)}}{250 \; \cancel{mL}} \right| \frac{}{50 \; \cancel{(kg)}} \left| \frac{25}{50} \right. = \frac{0.5 \; mg}{kg/hr}$$

CHAPTER 7

One-Factor Practice Problems

1. Sequential method:

$$\frac{200 \; \cancel{mg}}{} \left| \frac{\cancel{(mL)}}{100 \; \cancel{mg}} \right| \frac{2}{1} = 2 \; mL$$

○ **Chapter 7** continued

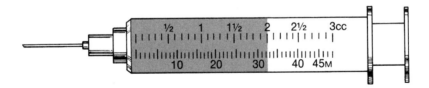

Problem example found in Chapter 4: One-Factor Medication Problems, Problem Example #2.

2. Sequential method:

$$\frac{30 \text{ mg} \boxed{\text{tablet}} 3}{|30 \text{ mg}|3} = 1 \text{ tablet}$$

Problem example found in Chapter 4: One Factor Medication Problems, Problem Example #2.

3. Sequential method:

$$\frac{7.5 \text{ mg} \boxed{\text{tablet}} 7.5}{|2.5 \text{ mg}|2.5} = 3 \text{ tablets}$$

Problem example found in Chapter 4: One-Factor Medication Problems, Drug Label Problem #3.

4. Sequential method:

$$\frac{160 \text{ mg} \mid 5 \text{ mL} \mid 1 \boxed{\text{tsp}} 1}{|160 \text{ mg}| 5 \text{ mL} \mid} = 1 \text{ tsp}$$

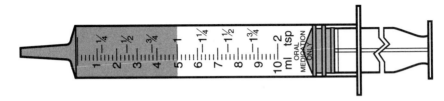

Problem example found in Chapter 4: One-Factor Medication Problems, Drug Label Problem #4.

5. Sequential method:

$$\frac{0.5 \; \text{mg} \; \boxed{\text{tablet}} \; 0.5}{1 \; \text{mg} \mid 1} = 0.5 \; \text{tablet}$$

Problem example found in Chapter 4: One-Factor Medication Problems, Drug Label Problem #4.

6. Sequential method:

$$\frac{60 \; \text{mg}}{} \left| \frac{\boxed{\text{tablet}}}{60 \; \text{mg}} \right. = 1 \; \text{tablet}$$

Problem example found in Chapter 4: One-Factor Medication Problems, Problem Example #2.

7. Sequential method:

$$\frac{0.25 \; \text{mg} \mid \boxed{\text{tablet}} \mid 0.25}{\mid 0.125 \; \text{mg} \mid 0.125} = 2 \; \text{tablets}$$

Problem example found in Chapter 4: One-Factor Medication Problems, Drug Label Problem #3.

8. Sequential method:

$$\frac{80 \; \text{mg} \; \boxed{\text{tablet}} \mid 8}{\mid 20 \; \text{mg} \mid 2} = 4 \; \text{tablets}$$

Problem example found in Chapter 4: One-Factor Medication Problems, Problem Example #2.

9. Random method:

$$\frac{10 \; \text{mg} \; \boxed{\text{mL}} \mid 1 \; \text{gr} \mid 1 \times 1 \mid 1 \mid 1}{\mid \frac{1}{8} \; \text{gr} \mid 60 \; \text{mg} \mid \frac{1}{8} \times \frac{6}{1} \mid \frac{6}{8} \mid 0.75} = 1.33 \; \text{or} \; 1.3 \; \text{mL}$$

○ **Chapter 7** continued

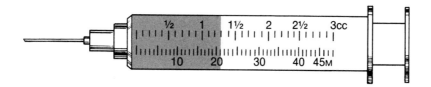

Problem example found in Chapter 4: One-Factor Medication Problems, Drug Label Problem #7.

10. Random method:

$$\frac{100 \text{ mcg} \mid \boxed{\text{mL}} \mid 1 \text{ mg} \mid 1 \times 1 \mid 1}{\mid 0.4 \text{ mg} \mid 1000 \text{ mcg} \mid 0.4 \times 10 \mid 4} = 0.25 \text{ or } 0.3 \text{ mL}$$

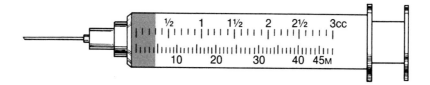

Problem example found in Chapter 4: One-Factor Medication Problems, Problem Example #3.

11. Sequential method:

$$\frac{80 \text{ mg} \mid 2 \boxed{\text{mL}} \mid 80 \times 2 \mid 160}{\mid 125 \text{ mg} \mid 125 \mid 125} = 1.28 \text{ or } 1.3 \text{ mL}$$

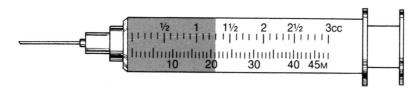

Problem example found in Chapter 4: One-Factor Medication Problems, Problem Example #1.

12. Sequential method:

$$\frac{20 \text{ gm} \, | \, 15 \, \boxed{\text{mL}} \, | \, 2 \times 15 \, | \, 30}{| \quad 10 \text{ g} \quad | \quad 1 \quad | \quad 1} = 30 \text{ mL}$$

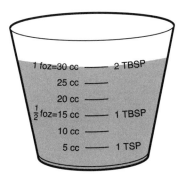

Problem example found in Chapter 4: One-Factor Medication Problems, Problem Example #1.

13. Sequential method:

$$\frac{5 \text{ mg} \quad | \quad \boxed{\text{mL}}}{| \quad 5 \text{ mg}} = 1 \text{ mL}$$

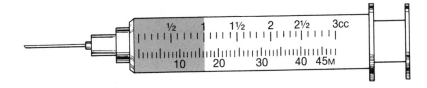

Problem example found in Chapter 4: One-Factor Medication Problems, Problem Example #1.

14. Sequential method:

$$\frac{250 \text{ mg} \, | \, 5 \, \boxed{\text{mL}} \, | \, 250 \times 5 \, | \, 1250}{| \quad 125 \text{ mg} \, | \quad 125 \quad | \quad 125} = 10 \text{ mL}$$

(Problem continues on next page)

○ **Chapter 7** continued

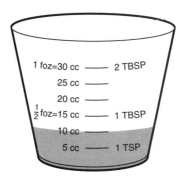

Problem example found in Chapter 4: One-Factor Medication Problems, Problem Example #1.

15. Sequential method:

$$\frac{200 \text{ mg} \left| \text{tablet} \right| 2}{\left| 100 \text{ mg} \right| 1} = 2 \text{ tablets}$$

Problem example found in Chapter 4: One-Factor Medication Problems, Problem Example #2.

16. Sequential method:

$$\frac{10 \text{ mg} \left| \text{tablet} \right| 10}{\left| 5 \text{ mg} \right| 5} = 2 \text{ tablets}$$

Problem example found in Chapter 4: One-Factor Medication Problems, Problem Example #1.

17. Sequential method:

$$\frac{3 \text{ mg} \left| \text{mL} \right| 3}{\left| 2 \text{ mg} \right| 2} = 1.5 \text{ mL}$$

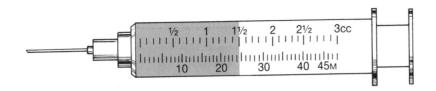

Problem example found in Chapter 4: One-Factor Medication Problems, Problem Example #1.

18. Sequential method:

$$\frac{400 \text{ mg}}{} \Bigg| \frac{10.15 \text{ (mL)}}{325 \text{ mg}} \Bigg| \frac{400 \times 10.15}{325} \Bigg| \frac{4060}{325} = 12.49 \text{ or } 12.5 \text{ mL}$$

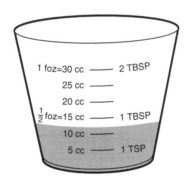

Problem example found in Chapter 4: One-Factor Medication Problems, Problem Example #1.

19. Random method:

$$\frac{1000 \text{ mg}}{} \Bigg| \frac{2 \text{ (mL)}}{1 \text{ g}} \Bigg| \frac{1 \text{ g}}{1000 \text{ mg}} \Bigg| \frac{2 \times 1}{1} \Bigg| \frac{2}{1} = 2 \text{ mL}$$

(Problem continues on next page)

○ **Chapter 7** continued

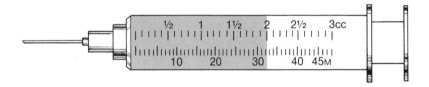

Problem example found in Chapter 4: One-Factor Medication Problems, Problem Example #3.

20. Random method:

$$\frac{10 \text{ mg}}{} \left| \frac{5 \text{ mL}}{5 \text{ mg}} \right| \frac{1 \text{ (tsp)}}{5 \text{ mL}} \left| \frac{10 \times 1}{5} \right| \frac{10}{5} = 2 \text{ tsp}$$

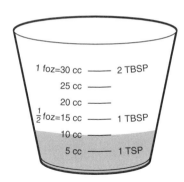

Problem example found in Chapter 4: One-Factor Medication Problems, Drug Label Problem #4.

Two-Factor Practice Problems

1. Random method:

$$\frac{25 \text{ mcg}}{\text{kg}} \left| \frac{2.5 \text{ (mL)}}{0.125 \text{ mg}} \right| \frac{1 \text{ kg}}{2.2 \text{ lb}} \left| \frac{1 \text{ mg}}{1000 \text{ mcg}} \right| \frac{25 \text{ lb}}{} = \text{mL}$$

$$\frac{25 \times 2.5 \times 1 \times 1 \times 25}{0.125 \times 2.2 \times 1000} \quad \Big| \quad \frac{1562.5 = 5.68 \text{ or } 5.7 \text{ mL}}{275}$$

Problem example found in Chapter 5: Two-Factor Medication Problems, Problem Example #1.

2. Sequential method:

$$\frac{0.2 \text{ mg}}{\text{kg}} \Big| \frac{\text{mL}}{0.1 \text{ mg}} \Big| \frac{1 \text{ kg}}{2.2 \text{ lb}} \Big| 35 \text{ lb} \Big| \frac{0.2 \times 1 \times 35}{0.1 \times 2.2} \Big| \frac{7}{0.22} = 3.18 \text{ or } 3.2 \text{ mL}$$

Problem example found in Chapter 5: Two-Factor Medication Problems, Problem Example #1.

3. Random method:

$$\frac{2 \text{ mg}}{\text{min}} \Big| \frac{500 \text{ mL}}{2 \text{ g}} \Big| \frac{1 \text{ g}}{1000 \text{ mg}} \Big| \frac{60 \text{ min}}{1 \text{ hr}} \Big| \frac{5 \times 6}{1} \Big| \frac{30}{1} = \frac{30 \text{ mL}}{\text{hr}}$$

Problem example found in Chapter 5: Two-Factor Medication Problems, Problem Example #7.

4. Sequential method:

$$\frac{1.5 \text{ g}}{} \Big| \frac{10 \text{ mL}}{1 \text{ g}} \Big| \frac{1.5 \times 10}{1} \Big| \frac{15}{1} = 15 \text{ mL}$$

Problem example found in Chapter 5: Two-Factor Medication Problems, Problem Example #3.

5. Sequential method:

$$\frac{1 \text{ mg}}{\text{kg}} \Big| \frac{\text{mL}}{40 \text{ mg}} \Big| \frac{1 \text{ kg}}{2.2 \text{ lb}} \Big| 94 \text{ lb} \Big| \frac{1 \times 1 \times 94}{40 \times 2.2} \Big| \frac{94}{88} = 1.068 \text{ or } 1.1 \text{ mL}$$

Problem example found in Chapter 5: Two-Factor Medication Problems, Problem Example #1.

◯ **Chapter 7** continued

6. Sequential method:

$$\frac{15 \text{ mg}}{\text{hr}} \left| \frac{500 \text{ mL}}{300 \text{ mg}} \right| \frac{15 \times 5}{3} \left| \frac{75}{3} \right. = 25 \frac{\text{mL}}{\text{hr}}$$

Problem example found in Chapter 5: Two-Factor Medication Problems, Problem Example #1.

7. Sequential method:

$$\frac{25 \text{ mL}}{\text{hr}} \left| \frac{50 \text{ mg}}{250 \text{ mL}} \right| 5 = 5 \frac{\text{mg}}{\text{hr}}$$

Problem example found in Chapter 5: Two-Factor Medication Problems, Problem Example #8.

8. Sequential method:

$$\frac{10 \text{ mEq}}{} \left| \frac{20 \text{ mL}}{20 \text{ mEq}} \right| 10 = 10 \text{ mL}$$

Problem example found in Chapter 5: Two-Factor Medication Problems, Problem Example #3.

9. Random method:

$$\frac{3 \text{ mL}}{\text{hr}} \left| \frac{50 \text{ mg}}{500 \text{ mL}} \right| \frac{1000 \text{ mcg}}{1 \text{ mg}} \left| \frac{1 \text{ hr}}{60 \text{ min}} \right| \frac{3 \times 10}{6} \left| \frac{30}{6} \right. = 5 \frac{\text{mcg}}{\text{min}}$$

Problem example found in Chapter 5: Two-Factor Medication Problems, Problem Example #8.

10. Sequential method:

$$\frac{100 \text{ mL}}{\text{hr}} \Bigg| \frac{10 \text{ (mEq)}}{1000 \text{ mL}} \Bigg| 1 = 1 \frac{\text{mEq}}{\text{hr}}$$

Problem example found in Chapter 5: Two-Factor Medication Problems, Problem Example #8.

11. Sequential method:

$$\frac{250 \text{ mL}}{\text{hr}} \Bigg| \frac{20 \text{ (gtt)}}{\text{mL}} \Bigg| \frac{1 \text{ hr}}{60 \text{ (min)}} \Bigg| \frac{250 \times 2 \times 1}{6} \Bigg| \frac{500}{6} = 83.3 \text{ or } 83 \frac{\text{gtt}}{\text{min}}$$

Problem example found in Chapter 5: Two-Factor Medication Problems, Problem Example #10.

12. Sequential method:

$$\frac{750 \text{ mL}}{5 \text{ hr}} \Bigg| \frac{10 \text{ (gtt)}}{\text{mL}} \Bigg| \frac{1 \text{ hr}}{60 \text{ (min)}} \Bigg| \frac{750 \times 1 \times 1}{5 \times 6} \Bigg| \frac{750}{30} = 25 \frac{\text{gtt}}{\text{min}}$$

Problem example found in Chapter 5: Two-Factor Medication Problems, Problem Example #10.

13. Sequential method:

$$\frac{500 \text{ mL}}{8 \text{ hr}} \Bigg| \frac{60 \text{ (gtt)}}{\text{mL}} \Bigg| \frac{1 \text{ hr}}{60 \text{ (min)}} \Bigg| \frac{500 \times 1}{8} \Bigg| \frac{500}{8} = 62.5 \text{ or } 63 \frac{\text{gtt}}{\text{min}}$$

Problem example found in Chapter 5: Two-Factor Medication Problems, Problem Example #10.

14. Sequential method:

$$\frac{750 \text{ mL}}{} \Bigg| \frac{15 \text{ gtt}}{\text{mL}} \Bigg| \frac{\text{min}}{18 \text{ gtt}} \Bigg| \frac{1 \text{ (hr)}}{60 \text{ min}} \Bigg| \frac{750 \times 15 \times 1}{18 \times 60} \Bigg| \frac{11250}{1080} = 10.41 \text{ or } 10 \text{ hr}$$

◯ **Chapter 7** continued

Problem example found in Chapter 5: Two-Factor Medication Problems, Problem Example #11.

15. Sequential method:

$$\frac{250 \text{ mL}}{} \Big| \frac{15 \text{ gtt}}{\text{mL}} \Big| \frac{\text{min}}{50 \text{ gtt}} \Big| \frac{1 \text{ (hr)}}{60 \text{ min}} \Big| \frac{25 \times 15 \times 1}{50 \times 6} \Big| \frac{375}{300} = 1.25 \text{ or } 1 \text{ hr}$$

Problem example found in Chapter 5: Two-Factor Medication Problems, Problem Example #11.

16. Sequential method:

$$\frac{1000 \text{ mL}}{} \Big| \frac{15 \text{ gtt}}{\text{mL}} \Big| \frac{\text{min}}{25 \text{ gtt}} \Big| \frac{1 \text{ (hr)}}{60 \text{ min}} \Big| \frac{100 \times 15 \times 1}{25 \times 6} \Big| \frac{1500}{150} = 10 \text{ hr}$$

Problem example found in Chapter 5: Two-Factor Medication Problems, Problem Example #11.

17. Sequential method:

$$\frac{1.25 \text{ g}}{} \Big| \frac{10 \text{ (mL)}}{1 \text{ gm}} \Big| \frac{1.25 \times 10}{1} \Big| \frac{12.5}{1} = 12.5 \text{ mL}$$

Calculate milliliter per hour to set the IV pump.
Sequential method:

$$\frac{112.5 \text{ (mL)}}{\text{(hr)}} = 112.5 \text{ or } \frac{113 \text{ mL}}{\text{hr}}$$

Calculate drops per minute with a drop factor of 10 gtt/mL.
Sequential method:

$$\frac{112.5 \text{ mL}}{\text{hr}} \Big| \frac{10 \text{ (gtt)}}{\text{mL}} \Big| \frac{1 \text{ hr}}{60 \text{ (min)}} \Big| \frac{112.5 \times 1 \times 1}{6} \Big| \frac{112.5}{6} = 18.75 \text{ or } 19 \frac{\text{gtt}}{\text{min}}$$

Problem example found in Chapter 5: Two-Factor Medication Problems, Problem Example #12.

18. How many milliliters will you draw from the vial after reconstitution?
Sequential method:

$$\frac{275 \text{ mg}}{} \bigg| \frac{10 \text{ (mL)}}{500 \text{ mg}} \bigg| \frac{275 \times 1}{50} \bigg| \frac{275}{50} = 5.5 \text{ mL}$$

Calculate milliliters per hour to set the IV pump.
Sequential method:

$$\frac{255.5 \text{ (mL)}}{\text{(hr)}} = 255.5 \text{ or } \frac{256 \text{ mL}}{\text{hr}}$$

Calculate drops per minute with a drop factor of 10 gtt/mL.
Sequential method:

$$\frac{255.5 \text{ mL}}{\text{hr}} \bigg| \frac{10 \text{ (gtt)}}{\text{mL}} \bigg| \frac{1 \text{ hr}}{60 \text{ (min)}} \bigg| \frac{255.5 \times 1 \times 1}{6} \bigg| \frac{255.5}{6} = 42.5 \text{ or } 43 \frac{\text{gtt}}{\text{min}}$$

Problem example found in Chapter 5: Two-Factor Medication Problems, Problem Example #12.

19. Random method:

$$\frac{450 \text{ mg}}{} \bigg| \frac{10 \text{ (mL)}}{1 \text{ g}} \bigg| \frac{1 \text{ g}}{1000 \text{ mg}} \bigg| \frac{45 \times 1}{10} \bigg| \frac{45}{10} = 4.5 \text{ mL}$$

Calculate milliliters per hour to set the IV pump.
Sequential method:

$$\frac{104.5 \text{ (mL)}}{30 \text{ min}} \bigg| \frac{60 \text{ min}}{1 \text{ (hr)}} \bigg| \frac{104.5 \times 6}{3 \times 1} \bigg| \frac{627}{3} = 209 \frac{\text{mL}}{\text{hr}}$$

◯ **Chapter 7** continued

Calculate drops per minute with a drop factor of 10 gtt/mL.
Sequential method:

$$\frac{104.5 \text{ mL}}{30 \text{ min}} \left| \frac{10 \text{ gtt}}{\text{mL}} \right| \frac{104.5 \times 1}{3} \left| \frac{104.5}{3} \right| = 34.8 \text{ or } 35 \frac{\text{gtt}}{\text{min}}$$

Problem example found in Chapter 5: Two-Factor Medication Problems, Problem
Example #12.

20. How many milliliters will you draw from the vial?
Sequential method:

$$\frac{23 \text{ mg}}{} \left| \frac{\text{mL}}{40 \text{ mg}} \right| \frac{23}{40} = 0.57 \text{ or } 0.6 \text{ mL}$$

Calculate milliliters per hour to set the IV pump.
Sequential method:

$$\frac{100.6 \text{ mL}}{\text{hr}} = 100.6 \text{ or } \frac{101 \text{ mL}}{\text{hr}}$$

Calculate drops per minute with a drop factor of 15 gtt/mL.

$$\frac{100.6 \text{ mL}}{\text{hr}} \left| \frac{15 \text{ gtt}}{\text{mL}} \right| \frac{1 \text{ hr}}{60 \text{ min}} \left| \frac{100.6 \times 15 \times 1}{60} \right| \frac{1509}{60} = 25.15 \text{ or } 25 \frac{\text{gtt}}{\text{min}}$$

Problem example found in Chapter 5: Two-Factor Medication Problems, Problem
Example #12.

Three-Factor Practice Problems

1. Sequential method:

$$\frac{40 \text{ mg}}{\text{kg/day}} \left| \frac{5 \text{ mL}}{300 \text{ mg}} \right| \frac{60 \text{ kg}}{} \left| \frac{4 \times 5 \times 6}{3} \right| \frac{120}{3} = 40 \frac{\text{mL}}{\text{day}}$$

How many milliliters per dose will you give?

Sequential method:

$$\frac{40 \text{ mg}}{\text{kg/day}} \left| \frac{5 \text{ (mL)}}{300 \text{ mg}} \right| \frac{60 \text{ kg}}{} \left| \frac{\text{day}}{4 \text{ (doses)}} \right| \frac{4 \times 5 \times 6}{3 \times 4} \left| \frac{120}{12} \right. = \frac{10 \text{ mL}}{\text{dose}}$$

Problem example found in Chapter 6: Three-Factor Medication Problems, Problem Example #1.

2. Sequential method:

$$\frac{4 \text{ mg}}{\text{kg/(day)}} \left| \frac{\text{(mL)}}{10 \text{ mg}} \right| \frac{1 \text{ kg}}{2.2 \text{ lb}} \left| \frac{60 \text{ lb}}{} \right| \frac{4 \times 1 \times 6}{1 \times 2.2} \left| \frac{24}{2.2} \right. = 10.9 \text{ or } \frac{11 \text{ mL}}{\text{day}}$$

Problem example found in Chapter 6: Three-Factor Medication Problems, Problem Example #1.

3. Sequential method:

$$\frac{30 \text{ mg}}{\text{kg/(day)}} \left| \frac{2 \text{ (mL)}}{300 \text{ mg}} \right| \frac{50 \text{ kg}}{} \left| \frac{2 \times 5}{} \right| \frac{10}{} = \frac{10 \text{ mL}}{\text{day}}$$

How many milliliters per dose will you give?
Sequential method:

$$\frac{30 \text{ mg}}{\text{kg/day}} \left| \frac{2 \text{ (mL)}}{300 \text{ mg}} \right| \frac{50 \text{ kg}}{} \left| \frac{\text{day}}{3 \text{ (doses)}} \right| \frac{2 \times 5}{3} \left| \frac{10}{3} \right. = 3.33 \text{ or } \frac{3.3 \text{ mL}}{\text{dose}}$$

Problem example found in Chapter 6: Three-Factor Medication Problems, Problem Example #1.

4. Sequential method:

$$\frac{0.575 \text{ mL}}{\text{dose}} \left| \frac{40 \text{ (mg)}}{\text{mL}} \right| \frac{2.2 \text{ lb}}{1 \text{ (kg)}} \left| \frac{}{45 \text{ lb}} \right| \frac{3 \text{ doses}}{\text{(day)}} = \frac{\text{mg}}{\text{kg/day}}$$

$$\frac{0.575 \times 40 \times 2.2 \times 3}{1 \times 45} \left| \frac{151.8}{45} \right. = 3.37 \text{ or } \frac{3.4 \text{ mg}}{\text{kg/day}}$$

Problem example found in Chapter 6: Three-Factor Medication Problems, Problem Example #2.

○ **Chapter 7** continued

5. Sequential method:

$$\frac{0.125 \text{ mL}}{\text{dose}} \left| \frac{50 \text{ (mg)}}{\text{mL}} \right| \frac{2.2 \text{ lb}}{1 \text{ (kg)}} \left| \frac{}{20 \text{ lb}} \right| \frac{3 \text{ doses}}{\text{(day)}} = \frac{\text{mg}}{\text{kg/day}}$$

$$\frac{0.125 \times 5 \times 2.2 \times 3}{1 \times 2} \quad \frac{4.125 = 2.06 \text{ or } 2.1}{2} \quad \frac{\text{mg}}{\text{kg/day}}$$

Problem example found in Chapter 6: Three-Factor Medication Problems, Problem Example #2.

6. Sequential method:

$$\frac{400 \text{ mg}}{} \left| \frac{10 \text{ (mL)}}{400 \text{ mg}} \right| 10 = 10 \text{ mL}$$

Calculate milliliter per hour to set the IV pump.
Random method:

$$\frac{5 \text{ mcg}}{\text{kg/min}} \left| \frac{260 \text{ (mL)}}{400 \text{ mg}} \right| \frac{1 \text{ mg}}{1000 \text{ mcg}} \left| \frac{1 \text{ kg}}{2.2 \text{ lb}} \right| \frac{110 \text{ lb}}{} \left| \frac{60 \text{ min}}{1 \text{ (hr)}} \right| = \frac{\text{mL}}{\text{hr}}$$

$$\frac{5 \times 26 \times 1 \times 11 \times 6}{4 \times 100 \times 2.2} \quad \frac{8580 = 9.75 \text{ or } 9.8}{880} \quad \frac{\text{mL}}{\text{hr}}$$

Problem example found in Chapter 6: Three-Factor Medication Problems, Problem Example #3.

7. Random method:

$$\frac{0.8 \text{ mcg}}{\text{kg/min}} \left| \frac{500 \text{ (mL)}}{50 \text{ mg}} \right| \frac{1 \text{ mg}}{1000 \text{ mcg}} \left| \frac{1 \text{ kg}}{2.2 \text{ lb}} \right| \frac{60 \text{ min}}{1 \text{ (hr)}} \left| 143 \text{ lb} \right| = \frac{\text{mL}}{\text{hr}}$$

$$\frac{0.8 \times 5 \times 1 \times 6 \times 143}{5 \times 10 \times 2.2} \quad \frac{3432}{110} = 31.2 \ \frac{mL}{hr}$$

Problem example found in Chapter 6: Three-Factor Medication Problems, Problem Example #3.

8. Random method:

$$\frac{68 \ mL}{hr} \left| \frac{50 \ mg}{250 \ mL} \right| \frac{1 \ hr}{60 \ (min)} \left| \frac{2.2 \ lb}{1 \ (kg)} \right| \frac{1000 \ (mcg)}{1 \ mg} \right| \frac{}{250 \ lb} = \frac{mcg}{kg/min}$$

$$\frac{68 \times 5 \times 1 \times 2.2 \times 10}{25 \times 6 \times 1 \times 1 \times 25} \quad \frac{7480}{3750} = 1.99 \ or \ 2 \ \frac{mcg}{kg/min}$$

Problem example found in Chapter 6: Three-Factor Medication Problems, Problem Example #4.

9. Random method:

$$\frac{30 \ mg}{kg/(day)} \left| \frac{1 \ kg}{2.2 \ lb} \right| 157 \ lb \left| \frac{1 \ (g)}{1000 \ mg} \right| \frac{3 \times 1 \times 157 \times 1}{2.2 \times 100} \left| \frac{471}{220} \right. = 2.14 \ or \ 2.1 \ \frac{g}{day}$$

Problem example found in Chapter 6: Three-Factor Medication Problems, Problem Example #2.

10. Random method:

$$\frac{0.01 \ (mL)}{kg/min} \left| \frac{1 \ kg}{2.2 \ lb} \right| 180 \ lb \left| \frac{60 \ min}{1 \ (hr)} \right| \frac{0.01 \times 1 \times 180 \times 60}{2.2 \times 1} \left| \frac{108}{2.2} \right. =$$

$$\frac{108}{2.2} = 49.09 \ or \ 49.1 \ \frac{mL}{hr}$$

Problem example found in Chapter 6: Three-Factor Medication Problems, Problem Example #3.

11. Random method:

$$\frac{28 \ mL}{hr} \left| \frac{400 \ mg}{250 \ mL} \right| \frac{}{15 \ (kg)} \left| \frac{1 \ hr}{60 \ (min)} \right| \frac{1000 \ (mcg)}{1 \ mg} = \frac{mcg}{kg/min}$$

○ **Chapter 7** continued

$$\frac{28 \times 4 \times 1 \times 1000}{25 \times 15 \times 6 \times 1} \left| \frac{112000}{2250} \right. = 49.77 \text{ or } 49.8 \frac{\text{mcg}}{\text{kg/min}}$$

Problem example found in Chapter 6: Three-Factor Medication Problems, Problem Example #4.

12. Random method:

$$\frac{3 \text{ mcg}}{\text{kg/min}} \left| \frac{\cancel{100} \cancel{(mL)}}{\cancel{100} \text{ mg}} \right| \frac{1 \text{ kg}}{2.2 \text{ lb}} \left| \frac{\cancel{60} \cancel{\text{min}}}{1 \cancel{(hr)}} \right| \frac{160 \text{ lb}}{} \left| \frac{1 \text{ mg}}{\cancel{1000} \text{ mcg}} \right. = \frac{\text{mL}}{\text{hr}}$$

$$\frac{3 \times 1 \times 6 \times 16 \times 1}{2.2 \times 1 \times 10} \left| \frac{288}{22} \right. = 13.09 \text{ or } 13.1 \frac{\text{mL}}{\text{hr}}$$

Problem example found in Chapter 6: Three-Factor Medication Problems, Problem Example #3.

13. Random method:

$$\frac{68 \text{ mL}}{\text{hr}} \left| \frac{50 \text{ mg}}{\cancel{250} \text{ mL}} \right| \frac{\cancel{1} \cancel{\text{hr}}}{60 \cancel{(min)}} \left| \frac{2.2 \text{ lb}}{1 \cancel{(kg)}} \right| \frac{\cancel{1000} \cancel{(mcg)}}{\cancel{1} \text{ mg}} \left| \frac{}{250 \text{ lb}} \right. = \frac{\text{mcg}}{\text{kg/min}}$$

$$\frac{68 \times 50 \times 1 \times 2.2}{25 \times 6 \times 1 \times 25} \left| \frac{7480}{3750} \right. = 1.99 \text{ or } 2 \frac{\text{mcg}}{\text{kg/min}}$$

Problem example found in Chapter 6: Three-Factor Medication Problems, Problem Example #4.

14. Random method:

$$\frac{1 \text{ mcg}}{\text{kg/min}} \left| \frac{250 \cancel{(mL)}}{50 \text{ mg}} \right| \frac{\cancel{1} \text{ kg}}{2.2 \text{ lb}} \left| \frac{\cancel{60} \cancel{\text{min}}}{\cancel{1} \cancel{(hr)}} \right| \frac{160 \text{ lb}}{} \left| \frac{\cancel{1} \text{ mg}}{\cancel{1000} \text{ mcg}} \right. = \frac{\text{mL}}{\text{hr}}$$

$$\frac{1 \times 25 \times 1 \times 6 \times 16}{50 \times 2.2} \quad \Big| \quad \frac{2400}{110} = 21.81 \text{ or } 21.8 \frac{\text{mL}}{\text{hr}}$$

Problem example found in Chapter 6: Three-Factor Medication Problems, Problem Example #3.

15. Random method:

$$\frac{2.5 \text{ mcg}}{\text{kg/min}} \Big| \frac{500 \text{ (mL)}}{400 \text{ mg}} \Big| \frac{65 \text{ kg}}{1 \text{ (hr)}} \Big| \frac{60 \text{ min}}{} \Big| \frac{1 \text{ mg}}{1000 \text{ mcg}} = \frac{\text{mL}}{\text{hr}}$$

$$\frac{2.5 \times 5 \times 65 \times 6 \times 1}{4 \times 1 \times 100} \quad \Big| \quad \frac{4875}{400} = 12.18 \text{ or } 12.2 \frac{\text{mL}}{\text{hr}}$$

Problem example found in Chapter 6: Three-Factor Medication Problems, Problem Example #3.

16. Random method:

$$\frac{15 \text{ mL}}{\text{hr}} \Big| \frac{2 \text{ mg}}{500 \text{ mL}} \Big| \frac{1 \text{ hr}}{60 \text{ (min)}} \Big| \frac{1}{20 \text{ (kg)}} \Big| \frac{1000 \text{ (mcg)}}{1 \text{ mg}} = \frac{\text{mcg}}{\text{kg/min}}$$

$$\frac{15 \times 2 \times 1 \times 1}{5 \times 6 \times 20 \times 1} \quad \Big| \quad \frac{30}{600} = 0.05 \frac{\text{mcg}}{\text{kg/min}}$$

Problem example found in Chapter 6: Three-Factor Medication Problems, Problem Example #4.

17. Random method:

$$\frac{5 \text{ mcg}}{\text{kg/(min)}} \Big| \frac{500 \text{ (mL)}}{400 \text{ mg}} \Big| \frac{70 \text{ kg}}{} \Big| \frac{1 \text{ mg}}{1000 \text{ mcg}} = \frac{\text{mL}}{\text{min}}$$

◯ **Chapter 7** continued

$$\frac{5 \times 5 \times 7 \times 1}{4 \times 100} \quad \bigg| \quad \frac{175}{400} = 0.4375 \text{ or } 0.44 \frac{\text{mL}}{\text{min}}$$

Problem example found in Chapter 6: Three-Factor Medication Problems, Problem Example #3.

18. How many milligrams per day is the child receiving?
    Sequential method:

$$\frac{40 \text{ (mg)}}{\text{kg/(day)}} \bigg| \frac{1 \text{ kg}}{2.2 \text{ lb}} \bigg| \frac{20 \text{ lb}}{} \bigg| \frac{40 \times 1 \times 20}{2.2} \bigg| \frac{800}{2.2} = 363.63 \text{ or } 363.6 \frac{\text{mg}}{\text{day}}$$

How many milligrams per dose is the child receiving?
Sequential method:

$$\frac{363.6 \text{ (mg)}}{\text{day}} \bigg| \frac{\text{day}}{3 \text{ (doses)}} \bigg| \frac{363.6}{3} = 121.2 \frac{\text{mg}}{\text{dose}}$$

How many milliliters will you draw from the vial after reconstitution?
Sequential method:

$$\frac{121.2 \text{ mg}}{} \bigg| \frac{10 \text{ (mL)}}{500 \text{ mg}} \bigg| \frac{121.2 \times 10}{500} \bigg| \frac{1212}{500} = 2.424 \text{ or } 2.4 \text{ mL}$$

Calculate milliliters per hour to set the IV pump.
Sequential method:

$$\frac{102.4 \text{ (mL)}}{60 \text{ min}} \bigg| \frac{60 \text{ min}}{1 \text{ (hr)}} \bigg| \frac{102.4}{1} = 102.4 \frac{\text{mL}}{\text{hr}}$$

Problem example found in Chapter 6: Three-Factor Medication Problems, Problem Example #1.

19. How many milligrams per dose is the child receiving?

Random method:

$$\frac{2 \; \textcircled{mg} \; \Big| 40 \; \cancel{kg}}{\cancel{kg}/\textcircled{dose}} \Big| \frac{2 \times 40}{} \Big| \frac{80}{} = \frac{80 \; mg}{dose}$$

How many milliliters will you draw from the vial?
Sequential method:

$$\frac{80 \; \cancel{mg} \; \Big| \textcircled{mL}}{\Big| 40 \; \cancel{mg}} \Big| \frac{8}{4} = 2 \; mL$$

Calculate milliliters per hour to set the IV pump.
Sequential method:

$$\frac{52 \; \textcircled{mL} \; \Big| 60 \; \cancel{min}}{30 \; \cancel{min} \Big| 1 \; \textcircled{hr}} \Big| \frac{52 \times 6}{3 \times 1} \Big| \frac{312}{3} = \frac{104 \; mL}{hr}$$

Problem example found in Chapter 6: Three-Factor Medication Problems, Problem Example #1.

20. How many milligrams per day is the child receiving?
    Sequential method:

$$\frac{25 \; \textcircled{mg} \; \Big| 25 \; \cancel{kg}}{\cancel{kg}/\textcircled{day}} \Big| \frac{25 \times 25}{} \Big| \frac{625}{} = \frac{625 \; mg}{day}$$

How many milligrams per dose is the child receiving?
Sequential method:

$$\frac{625 \; \textcircled{mg} \; \Big| \; \cancel{day}}{\cancel{day} \; \Big| 3 \; \textcircled{doses}} \Big| \frac{625}{3} = 208.33 \; or \; \frac{208.3 \; mg}{dose}$$

How many milliliters will you draw from the vial after reconstitution?

○ **Chapter 7** continued

Sequential method:

$$\frac{208.3 \text{ mg}}{} \left| \frac{10 \text{ (mL)}}{500 \text{ mg}} \right| \frac{208.3 \times 1}{50} \left| \frac{208.3}{50} \right. = 4.166 \text{ or } 4.2 \text{ mL}$$

Calculate milliliters per hour to set the IV pump.
Sequential method:

$$\frac{54.2 \text{ (mL)}}{30 \text{ min}} \left| \frac{60 \text{ min}}{1 \text{ (hr)}} \right| \frac{54.2 \times 6}{3 \times 1} \left| \frac{325.2}{3} \right. = \frac{108.4 \text{ mL}}{\text{hr}}$$

Problem example found in Chapter 6: Three-Factor Medication Problems, Problem
Example #1.

Comprehensive Post-Test

1. Sequential method:

$$\frac{0.125 \text{ mg}}{} \left| \frac{\text{(tablet)}}{0.25 \text{ mg}} \right| \frac{0.125}{0.25} = 0.5 \text{ tablet}$$

Answer: 0.5 tablet
Additional practice problems found in Chapter 4: One-Factor Medication Problems.

2. Random method:

$$\frac{0.5 \text{ g}}{} \left| \frac{\text{(tablet)}}{500 \text{ mg}} \right| \frac{1000 \text{ mg}}{1 \text{ g}} \left| \frac{0.5 \times 10}{5 \times 1} \right| \frac{5}{5} = 1 \text{ tablet}$$

Answer: 1 tablet
Additional practice problems found in Chapter 4: One-Factor Medication Problems.

3. Random method:

$$\frac{\frac{1}{150} \text{ gr}}{} \left| \frac{\text{(mL)}}{0.4 \text{ mg}} \right| \frac{60 \text{ mg}}{1 \text{ gr}} \left| \frac{\frac{1}{150} \times \frac{60}{1}}{0.4 \times 1} \right| \frac{\frac{60}{150}}{0.4} \left| \frac{0.4}{0.4} \right. = 1 \text{ mL}$$

Answer: 1 mL
Additional practice problems found in Chapter 4: One-Factor Medication Problems.

4. Sequential method:

$$\frac{2 \text{ mg}}{\text{kg}} \left| \frac{10 \text{ (mL)}}{500 \text{ mg}} \right| \frac{75 \text{ kg}}{} \left| \frac{2 \times 1 \times 75}{50} \right| \frac{150}{50} = 3 \text{ mL}$$

Answer: 3 mL
Additional practice problems found in Chapter 5: Two-Factor Medication Problems.

5. Random method:

$$\frac{10 \text{ gr}}{} \left| \frac{\text{(tablet)}}{325 \text{ mg}} \right| \frac{60 \text{ mg}}{1 \text{ gr}} \left| \frac{10 \times 60}{325 \times 1} \right| \frac{600}{325} = 1.8 \text{ or 2 tablets}$$

Answer: 2 tablets
Additional practice problems found in Chapter 4: One-Factor Medication Problems.

6. Sequential method:

$$\frac{50 \text{ mg}}{} \left| \frac{\text{(mL)}}{100 \text{ mg}} \right| \frac{5}{10} = 0.5 \text{ mL}$$

Answer: 0.5 mL
Additional practice problems found in Chapter 4: One-Factor Medication Problems.

7. Sequential method:

$$\frac{2 \text{ mg}}{\text{kg}} \left| \frac{5 \text{ (mL)}}{500 \text{ mg}} \right| \frac{1 \text{ kg}}{2.2 \text{ lb}} \left| \frac{100 \text{ lb}}{} \right| \frac{2 \times 5 \times 1 \times 1}{5 \times 2.2} \left| \frac{10}{11} \right| = 0.9 \text{ mL}$$

Answer: 0.9 mL
Additional practice problems found in Chapter 5: Two-Factor Medication Problems.

8. Sequential method:

$$\frac{1000 \text{ mL}}{12 \text{ hr}} \left| \frac{15 \text{ (gtt)}}{\text{mL}} \right| \frac{1 \text{ hr}}{60 \text{ (min)}} \left| \frac{100 \times 15 \times 1}{12 \times 6} \right| \frac{1500}{72} = 20.8 \text{ or } 21 \frac{\text{gtt}}{\text{min}}$$

◯ **Chapter 8** continued

Answer: 21 gtt/min
Additional practice problems found in Chapter 5: Two-Factor Medication Problems.

9. Sequential method:

$$\frac{500 \text{ mL} \mid 15 \text{ gtt} \mid \text{ min} \mid 1 \text{ (hr)}}{\mid \text{ mL} \mid 21 \text{ gtt} \mid 60 \text{ min}} \frac{50 \times 15 \times 1}{21 \times 6} \frac{750}{126} = 5.9 \text{ hr}$$

Answer: 5.9 hours
Additional practice problems found in Chapter 5: Two-Factor Medication Problems.

10. Sequential method:

$$\frac{1500 \text{ units} \mid 250 \text{ (mL)}}{\text{(hr)} \mid 25,000 \text{ units}} \frac{15 \times 25}{25} \frac{375}{25} = 15 \frac{\text{mL}}{\text{hr}}$$

Answer: 15 mL/hr
Additional practice problems found in Chapter 5: Two-Factor Medication Problems.

11. Random method:

$$\frac{4 \text{ mcg} \mid 250 \text{ (mL)} \mid 1 \text{ mg} \mid 60 \text{ min} \mid 1 \text{ kg} \mid 120 \text{ lb}}{\text{kg/min} \mid 400 \text{ mg} \mid 1000 \text{ mcg} \mid 1 \text{ (hr)} \mid 2.2 \text{ lb}} = \frac{\text{mL}}{\text{hr}}$$

$$\frac{4 \times 25 \times 1 \times 6 \times 1 \times 12}{40 \times 10 \times 1 \times 2.2} \mid \frac{7200}{880} = 8.1 \text{ or } 8 \frac{\text{mL}}{\text{hr}}$$

Answer: 8 mL/hr
Additional practice problems found in Chapter 6: Three-Factor Medication Problems.

12. Random method:

$$\frac{750 \text{ mg} \mid \text{(mL)} \mid 1 \text{ g}}{\mid 1 \text{ g} \mid 1000 \text{ mg}} \frac{75 \times 1}{1 \times 100} \frac{75}{100} = 0.75 \text{ or } 0.8 \text{ mL}$$

Answer: 0.8 mL
Additional practice problems found in Chapter 6: Three-Factor Medication Problems.

13. Sequential method:

$$\frac{1000 \text{ mL}}{} \left| \frac{15 \text{ gtt}}{\text{mL}} \right| \frac{\text{min}}{50 \text{ gtt}} \left| \frac{1 \text{ hr}}{60 \text{ min}} \right| \frac{10 \times 15 \times 1}{5 \times 6} \left| \frac{150}{30} \right. = 5 \text{ hr}$$

Answer: 5 hours
Additional practice problems found in Chapter 4: Two-Factor Medication Problems.

14. Sequential method:

$$\frac{8 \text{ units}}{\text{hr}} \left| \frac{250 \text{ mL}}{100 \text{ units}} \right| \frac{8 \times 25}{10} \left| \frac{200}{} \right. = \frac{20 \text{ mL}}{\text{hr}}$$

Answer: 20 mL/hr
Additional practice problems found in Chapter 4: Two-Factor Medication Problems.

15. Random method:

$$\frac{0.8 \text{ mcg}}{\text{kg/min}} \left| \frac{500 \text{ mL}}{50 \text{ mg}} \right| \frac{1 \text{ mg}}{1000 \text{ mcg}} \left| \frac{1 \text{ kg}}{2.2 \text{ lb}} \right| \frac{143 \text{ lb}}{} \left| \frac{60 \text{ min}}{1 \text{ hr}} \right. = \frac{\text{mL}}{\text{hr}}$$

$$\frac{0.8 \times 5 \times 1 \times 1 \times 143 \times 6}{5 \times 10 \times 2.2 \times 1} \left| \frac{3432}{110} \right. = 31.2 \text{ or } \frac{31 \text{ mL}}{\text{hr}}$$

Answer: 31 mL/hr
Additional practice problems found in Chapter 6: Three-Factor Medication Problems.

16. Sequential method:

$$\frac{500 \text{ mL}}{8 \text{ hr}} \left| \frac{10 \text{ gtt}}{\text{mL}} \right| \frac{1 \text{ hr}}{60 \text{ min}} \left| \frac{50 \times 10 \times 1}{8 \times 6} \right| \frac{500}{48} = 10.4 \text{ or } \frac{10 \text{ gtt}}{\text{min}}$$

Answer: 10 gtt/min
Additional practice problems found in Chapter 5: Two-Factor Medication Problems.

17. Random method:

$$\frac{2 \text{ mEq}}{100 \text{ mL}} \left| \frac{10 \text{ mL}}{20 \text{ mEq}} \right| \frac{500 \text{ mL}}{} \left| \frac{2 \times 1 \times 5}{1 \times 2} \right| \frac{10}{2} = 5 \text{ mL}$$

○ **Chapter 8** continued

Answer: 5 mL
Additional practice problems found in Chapter 6: Three-Factor Medication Problems.

18. Sequential method:

$$\frac{500{,}000 \ \cancel{units}}{} \left| \frac{\cancel{mL}}{100{,}000 \ \cancel{units}} \right| \frac{1 \ \boxed{tsp}}{5 \ \cancel{mL}} \right| \frac{5 \times 1}{1 \times 5} \Bigg| \frac{5}{5} = 1 \ tsp$$

Answer: 1 tsp
Additional practice problems found in Chapter 4: One-Factor Medication Problems.

19. Random method:

$$\frac{44 \ \cancel{mg}}{\boxed{hr}} \left| \frac{250 \ \boxed{mL}}{1 \ \cancel{g}} \right| \frac{1 \ \cancel{g}}{1000 \ \cancel{mg}} \right| \frac{44 \times 25 \times 1}{1 \times 100} \Bigg| \frac{1100}{100} = 11 \ \frac{mL}{hr}$$

Answer: 11 mL/hr
Additional practice problems found in Chapter 5: Two-Factor Medication Problems.

20. Sequential method:

$$\frac{140 \ \cancel{mL}}{\boxed{hr}} \left| \frac{30 \ \boxed{mg}}{1000 \ \cancel{mL}} \right| \frac{14 \times 3}{10} \Bigg| \frac{42}{10} = 4.2 \ \frac{mg}{hr}$$

Answer: 4.2 mg/hr
Additional practice problems found in Chapter 5: Two-Factor Medication Problems.

CHAPTER 9

Case Study A

1. $\dfrac{50 \ \cancel{cc}}{\cancel{hr}} \left| \dfrac{60 \ \boxed{gtt}}{\cancel{mL}} \right| \dfrac{1 \ \cancel{hr}}{60 \ \boxed{min}} \right| \dfrac{50 \times 1}{} = \dfrac{50 \ gtt}{min}$

2. $\dfrac{10 \ \cancel{lb}}{} \left| \dfrac{1 \ \boxed{kg}}{2.2 \ \cancel{lb}} \right| \dfrac{10}{2.2} = 4.5 \ kg$

3. $\dfrac{40 \ \cancel{mg}}{} \left| \dfrac{\boxed{mL}}{10 \ \cancel{mg}} \right| \dfrac{4}{1} = 4 \ mL$

4. $\dfrac{0.125 \ \cancel{mg}}{} \left| \dfrac{\boxed{tablet}}{0.25 \ \cancel{mg}} \right| \dfrac{0.125}{0.25} = 0.5 \ tablet$

5. $\dfrac{20 \ \cancel{mEq}}{} \left| \dfrac{\boxed{tablet}}{10 \ \cancel{mEq}} \right| \dfrac{2}{1} = 2 \ tablets$

Case Study B

1. $\dfrac{1000 \text{ ⓒⓒ}}{8 \text{ ⓗⓡ}} \bigg| \dfrac{1000}{8} = \dfrac{125 \text{ cc}}{\text{hr}}$

2. $\dfrac{5.6 \text{ mg}}{\text{kg/30 min}} \bigg| \dfrac{100 \text{ ⓒⓒ}}{100 \text{ mg}} \bigg| \dfrac{1 \text{ kg}}{2.2 \text{ lb}} \bigg| \dfrac{140 \text{ lb}}{} \bigg| \dfrac{60 \text{ min}}{1 \text{ ⓗⓡ}} \bigg| \dfrac{5.6 \times 14 \times 6}{3 \times 2.2} \bigg| \dfrac{470.4}{6.6} = \dfrac{71.3 \text{ cc}}{\text{hr}}$

3. $\dfrac{0.5 \text{ mg}}{\text{kg/ⓗⓡ}} \bigg| \dfrac{250 \text{ ⓒⓒ}}{1 \text{ gm}} \bigg| \dfrac{1 \text{ gm}}{1000 \text{ mg}} \bigg| \dfrac{1 \text{ kg}}{2.2 \text{ lb}} \bigg| \dfrac{140 \text{ lb}}{} \bigg| \dfrac{0.5 \times 25 \times 1 \times 14}{10 \times 2.2} \bigg| \dfrac{175}{22} = \dfrac{7.9 \text{ cc}}{\text{hr}}$

4. $\dfrac{800 \text{ mg}}{} \bigg| \dfrac{20 \text{ ⓒⓒ}}{1 \text{ gm}} \bigg| \dfrac{1 \text{ gm}}{1000 \text{ mg}} \bigg| \dfrac{8 \times 2}{1} = 16 \text{ mL}$

   $\dfrac{266 \text{ ⓜⓁ}}{1 \text{ ⓗⓡ}} = \dfrac{266 \text{ cc}}{\text{hr}}$

5. $\dfrac{3 \text{ L}}{\text{day}} \bigg| \dfrac{\text{day}}{3 \text{ ⓢⓗⓘⓕⓣⓢ}} \bigg| \dfrac{1000 \text{ ⓜⓁ}}{1 \text{ L}} \bigg| \dfrac{1000}{1} = \dfrac{1000 \text{ mL}}{\text{shift}}$

Case Study C

1. $\dfrac{125 \text{ cc}}{\text{hr}} \bigg| \dfrac{20 \text{ ⓖⓣⓣ}}{\text{mL}} \bigg| \dfrac{1 \text{ hr}}{60 \text{ ⓜⓘⓝ}} \bigg| \dfrac{125 \times 2 \times 1}{6} \bigg| \dfrac{250}{6} = \dfrac{41.6 \text{ or } 42 \text{ gtt}}{\text{min}}$

2. $\dfrac{5 \text{ ⓜⓒⓖ}}{\text{kg}} \bigg| \dfrac{1 \text{ kg}}{2.2 \text{ lb}} \bigg| \dfrac{160 \text{ lb}}{} \bigg| \dfrac{5 \times 1 \times 160}{2.2} \bigg| \dfrac{800}{2.2} = \dfrac{363.6 \text{ mcg}}{}$

3. $\dfrac{80 \text{ mg}}{} \bigg| \dfrac{\text{ⓜⓁ}}{40 \text{ mg}} \bigg| \dfrac{8}{4} = 2 \text{ mL}$

   $\dfrac{102 \text{ ⓒⓒ}}{1 \text{ ⓗⓡ}} = \dfrac{102 \text{ cc}}{\text{hr}}$

4. $\dfrac{8 \text{ mg}}{} \bigg| \dfrac{\text{ⓜⓁ}}{4 \text{ mg}} \bigg| \dfrac{8}{4} = 2 \text{ mL}$

5. $\dfrac{50 \text{ ⓜⓁ}}{30 \text{ min}} \bigg| \dfrac{60 \text{ min}}{1 \text{ ⓗⓡ}} \bigg| \dfrac{50 \times 6}{3 \times 1} \bigg| \dfrac{300}{3} = \dfrac{100 \text{ cc}}{\text{hr}}$

Case Study D

1. $\dfrac{150 \text{ cc}}{\text{hr}} \bigg| \dfrac{20 \text{ ⓖⓣⓣ}}{\text{mL}} \bigg| \dfrac{1 \text{ hr}}{60 \text{ min}} \bigg| \dfrac{150 \times 20 \text{ gtts} \times 1}{6} \bigg| \dfrac{150}{6} = 50 \text{ gtts/min}$

2. $\dfrac{350 \text{ mg}}{} \bigg| \dfrac{10 \text{ ⓜⓁ}}{500 \text{ mg}} \bigg| \dfrac{35 \times 1}{5} \bigg| \dfrac{35}{5} = 7 \text{ mL}$

   107 cc/1 hr = 107 cc/hr

3. $\dfrac{300 \text{ mcg}}{} \bigg| \dfrac{1 \text{ ⓜⓁ}}{300 \text{ mcg}} = 1 \text{ mL}$

4. $\dfrac{100 \text{ units}}{\text{kg}} \bigg| \dfrac{\text{ⓜⓁ}}{4000 \text{ units}} \bigg| \dfrac{1 \text{ kg}}{2.2 \text{ lb}} \bigg| \dfrac{100 \text{ lb}}{} \bigg| \dfrac{10 \times 1 \times 1}{4 \times 2.2} \bigg| \dfrac{10}{8.8} = 1.1 \text{ mL}$

5. $\dfrac{800 \text{ mg}}{} \bigg| \dfrac{10 \text{ ⓜⓁ}}{1 \text{ gm}} \bigg| \dfrac{1 \text{ gm}}{1000 \text{ mg}} \bigg| \dfrac{80 \times 1}{10} \bigg| \dfrac{80}{10} = 8 \text{ mL}$

   $\dfrac{108 \text{ ⓜⓁ}}{60 \text{ min}} \bigg| \dfrac{60 \text{ min}}{1 \text{ ⓗⓡ}} \bigg| \dfrac{108}{1} = \dfrac{108 \text{ cc}}{\text{hr}}$

Case Study E

1. $\dfrac{150 \text{ cc}}{\text{hr}} \Big| \dfrac{10 \text{ gtt}}{\text{mL}} \Big| \dfrac{1 \text{ hr}}{60 \text{ min}} \Big| \dfrac{150 \times 1 \times 1}{6} \Big| \dfrac{150}{6} = \dfrac{25 \text{ gtt}}{\text{min}}$

2. $\dfrac{50 \text{ cc}}{15 \text{ min}} \Big| \dfrac{60 \text{ min}}{1 \text{ hr}} \Big| \dfrac{50 \times 60}{15 \times 1} \Big| \dfrac{3000}{15} = \dfrac{200 \text{ cc}}{\text{hr}}$

3. $\dfrac{5 \text{ mg}}{} \Big| \dfrac{\text{mL}}{10 \text{ mg}} \Big| \dfrac{5}{10} = 0.5 \text{ mL}$

4. $\dfrac{10 \text{ mg}}{\text{kg/day}} \Big| \dfrac{1 \text{ kg}}{2.2 \text{ lb}} \Big| \dfrac{125 \text{ lb}}{} \Big| \dfrac{10 \times 1 \times 125}{2.2} \Big| \dfrac{1250}{2.2} = \dfrac{568 \text{ mg}}{\text{day}}$

5. $\dfrac{0.5 \text{ mg}}{} \Big| \dfrac{\text{tablet}}{1 \text{ mg}} \Big| \dfrac{0.5}{1} = 0.5 \text{ tablet}$

Case Study F

1. $\dfrac{50 \text{ cc}}{\text{hr}} \Big| \dfrac{60 \text{ gtt}}{\text{mL}} \Big| \dfrac{1 \text{ hr}}{60 \text{ min}} \Big| \dfrac{50 \times 1}{} \Big| \dfrac{50}{} = \dfrac{50 \text{ gtt}}{\text{min}}$

2. $\dfrac{5000 \text{ units}}{} \Big| \dfrac{\text{mL}}{10,000 \text{ units}} \Big| \dfrac{5}{10} = 0.5 \text{ mL}$

3. $\dfrac{1000 \text{ units}}{\text{hr}} \Big| \dfrac{250 \text{ mL}}{25,000 \text{ units}} \Big| \dfrac{10}{} = \dfrac{10 \text{ mL}}{\text{hr}}$

4. $\dfrac{20 \text{ mg}}{} \Big| \dfrac{\text{mL}}{10 \text{ mg}} \Big| \dfrac{2}{1} = 2 \text{ mL}$

5. $\dfrac{5 \text{ mg}}{} \Big| \dfrac{\text{mL}}{10 \text{ mg}} \Big| \dfrac{5}{10} = 0.5 \text{ mL}$

Case Study G

1. $\dfrac{80 \text{ cc}}{\text{hr}} \Big| \dfrac{20 \text{ mEq}}{1 \text{ L}} \Big| \dfrac{1 \text{ L}}{1000 \text{ mL}} \Big| \dfrac{8 \times 2}{10} \Big| \dfrac{16}{10} = \dfrac{1.6 \text{ mEq}}{\text{hr}}$

2. $\dfrac{2 \text{ gm}}{} \Big| \dfrac{10 \text{ mL}}{2 \text{ gm}} \Big| \dfrac{10}{} = 10 \text{ mL}$

$\dfrac{60 \text{ cc}}{30 \text{ min}} \Big| \dfrac{60 \text{ min}}{1 \text{ hr}} \Big| \dfrac{60 \times 6}{3 \times 1} \Big| \dfrac{360}{3} = \dfrac{120 \text{ cc}}{\text{hr}}$

3. $\dfrac{1 \text{ gm}}{} \Big| \dfrac{10 \text{ mL}}{500 \text{ mg}} \Big| \dfrac{1000 \text{ mg}}{1 \text{ gm}} \Big| \dfrac{10 \times 10}{5} \Big| \dfrac{100}{5} = 20 \text{ mL}$

$\dfrac{120 \text{ mL}}{60 \text{ min}} \Big| \dfrac{60 \text{ min}}{1 \text{ hr}} \Big| \dfrac{120}{1} = \dfrac{120 \text{ cc}}{\text{hr}}$

4. $\dfrac{1 \text{ gm}}{} \Big| \dfrac{4 \text{ mL}}{600 \text{ mg}} \Big| \dfrac{1000 \text{ mg}}{1 \text{ gm}} \Big| \dfrac{4 \times 10}{6} \Big| \dfrac{40}{6} = 6.7 \text{ mL}$

$\dfrac{107 \text{ mL}}{1 \text{ hr}} \Big| \dfrac{107}{1} = \dfrac{107 \text{ mL}}{\text{hr}}$

5. $\dfrac{800 \text{ mg}}{} \Big| \dfrac{20 \text{ mL}}{1 \text{ gm}} \Big| \dfrac{1 \text{ gm}}{1000 \text{ mg}} \Big| \dfrac{8 \times 2}{1} \Big| \dfrac{16}{1} = 16 \text{ ml}$

$\dfrac{266 \text{ mL}}{60 \text{ min}} \Big| \dfrac{60 \text{ min}}{1 \text{ hr}} \Big| \dfrac{266}{1} = \dfrac{266 \text{ mL}}{\text{hr}}$

Case Study H

1. $\dfrac{400\ \text{mg}}{}\bigg|\dfrac{4\ \text{mL}}{600\ \text{mg}}\bigg|\dfrac{4 \times 4}{6}\bigg|\dfrac{16}{6} = 2.7\ \text{mL}$

   $\dfrac{53\ \text{mL}}{\text{hr}}\bigg|\ \dfrac{53}{} = \dfrac{53\ \text{cc}}{\text{hr}}$

2. $\dfrac{53\ \text{cc}}{\text{hr}}\bigg|\dfrac{20\ \text{gtt}}{\text{mL}}\bigg|\dfrac{1\ \text{hr}}{60\ \text{min}}\bigg|\dfrac{53 \times 2 \times 1}{6}\bigg|\dfrac{106}{6} = \dfrac{18\ \text{gtt}}{\text{min}}$

3. $\dfrac{200\ \text{mg}}{}\bigg|\dfrac{\text{tsp}}{30\ \text{mg}}\bigg|\dfrac{5\ \text{cc}}{1\ \text{tsp}}\bigg|\dfrac{20 \times 5}{3 \times 1}\bigg|\dfrac{100}{3} = 33\ \text{cc}$

4. $\dfrac{2.5\ \text{mg}}{}\bigg|\dfrac{\text{tablet}}{5\ \text{mg}}\bigg|\dfrac{2.5}{5} = 0.5\ \text{tablet}$

5. $\dfrac{30\ \text{mg}}{}\bigg|\dfrac{\text{tablet}}{30\ \text{mg}}\bigg|\dfrac{30}{30} = 1\ \text{tablet}$

Case Study I

1. $\dfrac{60\ \text{cc}}{\text{hr}}\bigg|\dfrac{20\ \text{mEq}}{1\ \text{L}}\bigg|\dfrac{1\ \text{L}}{1000\ \text{mL}}\bigg|\dfrac{6 \times 2}{10}\bigg|\dfrac{12}{10} = \dfrac{1.2\ \text{mEq}}{\text{hr}}$

2. $\dfrac{21\ \text{cc}}{\text{hr}}\bigg|\dfrac{25\ \text{mg}}{500\ \text{cc}}\bigg|\dfrac{21 \times 25}{500}\bigg|\dfrac{525}{500} = \dfrac{1.05\ \text{mg}}{\text{hr}}$

3. $\dfrac{21\ \text{cc}}{\text{hr}}\bigg|\dfrac{50\ \text{mg}}{500\ \text{cc}}\bigg|\dfrac{21 \times 5}{50}\bigg|\dfrac{105}{50} = \dfrac{2.1\ \text{mg}}{\text{hr}}$

4. $\dfrac{11\ \text{cc}}{\text{hr}}\bigg|\dfrac{25,000\ \text{units}}{250\ \text{cc}}\bigg|\dfrac{11 \times 2500}{25}\bigg|\dfrac{27500}{25} = \dfrac{1100\ \text{units}}{\text{hr}}$

5. $\dfrac{2\ \text{mg}}{}\bigg|\dfrac{\text{mL}}{0.25\ \text{mg}}\bigg|\dfrac{2}{0.25} = 8\ \text{mL}$

Case Study J

1. $\dfrac{125\ \text{cc}}{\text{hr}}\bigg|\dfrac{20\ \text{gtt}}{\text{mL}}\bigg|\dfrac{1\ \text{hr}}{60\ \text{min}}\bigg|\dfrac{125 \times 2 \times 1}{6}\bigg|\dfrac{250}{6} = \dfrac{41.66\ \text{gtt}}{\text{min}}$

2. $\dfrac{11\ \text{cc}}{\text{hr}}\bigg|\dfrac{150\ \text{mg}}{250\ \text{cc}}\bigg|\dfrac{11 \times 15}{25}\bigg|\dfrac{165}{25} = \dfrac{6.6\ \text{mg}}{\text{hr}}$

3. $\dfrac{10\ \text{mg}}{}\bigg|\dfrac{\text{mL}}{10\ \text{mg}}\bigg|\dfrac{10}{10} = 1\ \text{mL}$

4. $\dfrac{50\ \text{mg}}{}\bigg|\dfrac{\text{tablet}}{25\ \text{mg}}\bigg|\dfrac{50}{25} = 2\ \text{tablets}$

5. $\dfrac{80\ \text{mg}}{}\bigg|\dfrac{\text{mL}}{10\ \text{mg}}\bigg|\dfrac{8}{1} = 8\ \text{mL}$

Page numbers followed by *f* indicate figures; those followed by *t* indicate tabular material.

A

Abbreviation symbols, in prescriptions, 28*t*–31*t*, 32–34

Acetaminophen, dosage calculation for, 139, 139*f*, 146, 146*f*

Adalat (nifedipine), dosage calculation for, 140, 140*f*

Alprazolam (Xanax), dosage calculation for, 65, 65*f*, 139, 139*f*

Aminophylline, intravenous, dosage calculation for, 101–104

Amoxicillin/clavulanate (Augmentin), dosage calculation for, 83, 83*f*, 144, 144*f*

Ancef (cefazolin)
    for children, weight and, 129*f*, 129–130
    intravenous, for children, reconstitution of, 158, 158*f*
    reconstitution of, 97, 97*f*

Apothecary measurement system, 30, 30*t*–31*t*, 32
    abbreviations for, 30*t*
    conversion to other systems, 31*t*
    definition of, 201
    Roman numerals in, 2–11

Arabic numbers, 2–11, 22–23

Arithmetic, for calculation of drug dosage, review of, 1–26

Atropine sulfate, dosage calculation for, 78, 78*f*, 90–91, 91*f*
    for children, 149, 149*f*

Augmentin (amoxicillin/clavulanate), dosage calculation for, 83, 83*f*, 144, 144*f*

B

Bretylium tosylate, intravenous, weight and, 133, 133*f*–134*f*

C

Caplets, administration of, 67, 67*f*

Capsules, administration of, 67, 67*f*

Carbamazepine (Tegretol), dosage calculation for, for liquid administration, 70*f*, 70–71

Cefazolin (Ancef). *See* Ancef (cefazolin)

Cefotaxime (Claforan), reconstitution of, calculations for, 95*f*, 95–96

Chemical names, on drug labels, 61

Children, dosage for, weight and, 117–123

Cimetidine (Tagamet). *See* Tagamet (cimetidine)

Ciprofloxacin (Cipro), dosage calculation for, 62*f*

Claforan (cefotaxime), reconstitution of, 95*f*, 95–96

Clindamycin (cleocin), dosage calculation for, in children, 131, 131*f*, 154, 154*f*

Common equivalents, 27–36

Compazine (prochlorperazine), dosage calculation for
    for injection, 74*f*, 74–75, 84, 144, 144*f*
    for liquid administration, 69, 69*f*, 147–148, 148*f*
    tablets, 64*f*, 64–65

Conversion factors
    definition of, 38, 201
    in dimensional analysis, 41
        one-factor problems for, 53–60
    in dosage calculations, 117–134, 129*f*–134*f*
        weight and, 85–92
    in drop factors, 104–110
    for intravenous medications, 98–104
    in medication reconstitution, 93–98

D

Decimals, 17–26
    conversion to, from fractions, 15–17, 24–25
    division of, 18–19, 21, 26
    multiplication of, 18, 20, 25–26
    rounding of, 18, 19–20

Denominator
    definition of, 11, 201
    in dimensional analysis, 39, 41, 43
    in dosage calculation, 117–134, 129*f*–134*f*
        weight and, 85–92

Denominator (*continued*)
  in drop factors, 105
  in intermittent infusion, 111–116
  in intravenous medication administration, 98–104
  in reconstitution, 93–98
Digoxin, dosage calculation for, for elixir, 148, 148*f*
Diluents
  definition of, 201
  in reconstitution, 93, 96
Dimensional analysis
  in common equivalents, 27
  definition of, 38, 201
  in dosage calculation, 11, 15, 117–134, 129*f*–134*f*
    for infants and children, 85–92, 90*f*–93*f*
  in dosage calculations, weight and, 85–92
  and drop factors, in intravenous medication
    administration, 104–110
  in intermittent infusion, 111–116
  in one-factor medication problems, 53–84, 137–
    148
  in reconstitution, 93–98
  solving problems with, 37–50
  steps of, 39–41
  in three-factor medication problems, 153*f*–155*f*,
    153–158, 158*f*
  in two-factor medication problems, 148*f*–149*f*,
    148–152
Dipyradimole (Persantine), drug label for, and
    dosage, 82, 82*f*
Dividing line, 11
Dopamine, intravenous, dosage calculation for, 154–
    155, 155*f*
  by weight, 131, 131*f*–132*f*
Dosage
  arithmetic needed for, 1–26
  on drug labels, 61
  identification of, in medication orders, 52–53
  for infants and children, body weight and, 85–92,
    90*f*–93*f*
  measurement systems for, 27–32. *See also*
    Apothecary measurement system
  apothecary, 30, 30*t*–31*t*, 32
  household, 31*t*, 32

  metric, 28*f*–29*f*, 28*t*–29*t*, 28–29, 32. *See also*
    Metric system
  titration and, 117–118, 126–128
  weight and, for children, 117–123
Drop factors
  definition of, 201
  in intravenous medication administration, 104–
    110, 105*f*, 167
Drug dosage. *See* Dosage
Drug labels
  components of, 61
  definition of, 201
  and dosage calculations, 137–148, 138*f*–148*f*
  one-factor problems using, 62–66
    route of administration and, 68–84
  and reconstitution, 95*f*–97*f*, 95–97
Drugs
  administration of, five rights of, 1, 51–52
  forms of, on labels, 61
  identification of, in medication orders, 52–53

E

Enteric-coated medications
  administration of, 67, 67*f*
  definition of, 201
Equivalents, common, 27–36
Erythromycin, intravenous, reconstitution of, 111–112
Expiration date, on drug labels, 61

F

Factors, conversion. *See* Conversion factors
Fractions, 11–15
  conversion of, to decimals, 15–17, 24–25
  definition of, 201
  division of, 12–13, 14–15, 24
  multiplication of, 12, 13, 23
Furosemide, dosage calculation for, 90, 90*f*, 141,
    141*f*
  in children, 153, 153*f*
    by weight, 128–129, 129*f*

G

Generic names, on drug labels, 61
Given quantity
    definition of, 38, 202
    in dimensional analysis, 39–49, 62–66, 68–84
        one-factor problems for, 53–60
    in dosage calculation
        time and, 117–134, 129f–134f
        weight and, 85–92
    in drop factors, 104–110
    for intravenous medications, 98–104
    in reconstitution, 93–98
        for intermittent infusion, 111–116
Gravity flow
    definition of, 202
    in intravenous medication administration, 104

H

Halcion (triazolam), dosage calculation for, 63f, 63–64, 140, 140f
Heparin, intravenous, dosage calculation for, 99, 103–104
Household measurement system, 31t, 32, 202
Hydromorphone (Dilaudid), dosage calculation for, for injection, 79, 79f, 146–147, 147f

I

Infusion rate
    drop factor and, 104–110
    intermittent, calculation of, 111–116
Inserts, in packaging, use of for reconstitution, 94f, 94–95
Intermittent infusion
    definition of, 202
    reconstitution for, calculations for, 111–116
Intravenous medications
    administration of
        drop factors in, 104–110
        gravity flow in, 104

    intermittent infusion of, calculations for, 111–116
    reconstitution of, 96
    titration of, 117–118, 126–128
    tubing for, drop factors and, 104–110, 105f
    via pumps, calculations for, 98–104

L

Labels, for drugs. See Drug labels
Lactulose, dosage calculation for, 143, 143f
Lente human insulin (Novolin), dosage calculation for, 76–77, 77f
Liquid medications, administration of, 67, 67f, 68–84
Lot number, on drug labels, 61

M

Macrotubing, for gravity flow, 104, 105f
Magnesium sulfate, dosage calculation for, 147, 147f
Manufacturer, on drug labels, 61
Measurement systems, for dosage. See Dosage, measurement systems for
Medication cup, 67–72, 83
Medication orders, interpretation of, 52
Medication problems
    one-factor, 51–84
    three-factor, 117–134
    two-factor, 85–114
Medications. See Drugs; specific medications
Meperidine (Demerol), dosage calculation for, for intravenous administration, 79f, 79–80
Methylprednisolone (Solu-Medrol)
    dosage calculation for, for injection, 142, 142f
    reconstitution of, 94f, 94–95
Metolazone (Zaroxolyn), dosage calculation for, 84–85, 85f
Metric system, 28t–29t, 28–29, 32
    conversion to other systems, 31t
    definition of, 202
    household measurement equivalents for, 31t
    weight equivalents in, 28t

Mezlocillin (Mezlin), dosage calculation for, 149, 149*f*

Microtubing, for gravity flow, 104

Morphine sulfate, dosage calculation for, 138, 138*f*
    for injection, 91, 91*f*, 141, 141*f*
    for liquid administration, 75, 75*f*

N

Naloxone, dosage calculation for, for injection, 142, 142*f*

Nifedipine (Adalat), dosage calculation for, 140, 140*f*

Novolin (Lente human insulin), dosage calculation for, 76–77, 77*f*

NPH human insulin (Novolin), dosage calculation for, 76, 76*f*

Numerator
    definition of, 11, 202
    in dimensional analysis, 39, 41, 43
    in dosage calculation, weight and, 85–92, 117–134, 129*f*–134*f*
    in drop factors, 105
    in intermittent infusion, 111–116
    in intravenous medication administration, 98–104
    in reconstitution, 93–98

O

One-factor medication problems, 51–84, 62–66, 68–84, 137–148, 138*f*–148*f*, 202

Oral (PO) medications, administration of, 67

Orders, interpretation of, 52

Orinase (tolbutamide), dosage calculation for, 81, 81*f*

P

Package inserts, and reconstitution, 94*f*, 94–95

Parenteral administration, syringes for, 73*f*, 73–84

Patient, identification of, in medication orders, 52–53

Pediapred (prednisolone sodium phosphate), dosage calculation for, by weight, 130, 130*f*

Persantine (dipyridamole), dosage calculation for, 82, 82*f*

PO (oral) medications, administration of, 67

Powders, reconstitution of, calculations for, 86, 93–98, 94*f*–95*f*, 97*f*

Prednisolone sodium phosphate (Pediapred), dosage calculation for, by weight, 130, 130*f*

Prednisone, dosage calculation for, 138, 138*f*
    for tablets, 145, 145*f*

Prescriptions
    apothecary abbreviations in, 30, 30*t*–31*t*, 32
    five rights of, 51–52
    household abbreviations in, 31*t*, 32
    metric abbreviations in, 28*f*–29*f*, 28*t*–29*t*, 28–29, 32

Prochlorperazine (Compazine). *See* Compazine (prochlorperazine)

Pumps, intravenous, 98–104

Q

Quantity
    given. *See* Given quantity
    wanted. *See* Wanted quantity

R

Random method, of dimensional analysis, 53, 59, 202. *See also* Dimensional analysis

Reconstitution
    drug label information for, 95*f*–97*f*, 95–97
    for intermittent infusion, 111–116
    package insert information for, 94*f*, 94–95
    of powders, 86, 93–98, 94*f*–95*f*, 97*f*

Roman numerals, 2–11, 22–23

Route of administration, 68–84
    identification of, in medication orders, 52–53
    types of, 67

S

Sequential method, of dimensional analysis, 53, 55, 202. *See also* Dimensional Analysis
Solu-Medrol (methylprednisolone)
    dosage calculation for, for injection, 142, 142*f*
    reconstitution of, 94*f*, 94–95
Syringes, for drug administration, 67–72, 83
    parenteral, 73*f*, 73–84

T

Tablets, administration of, 67, 67*f*
Tagamet (cimetidine)
    administration of, as liquid, 68, 68*f*
    dosage calculation for, in children, 92, 92*f*, 153, 153*f*
    drug label for, components of, 61*f*
Tegretol (carbamazepine), dosage calculation for, for liquid administration, 70*f*, 70–71
Three-factor medication problems, 117–134, 153*f*–155*f*, 153–158, 158*f*, 202
Tigan (trimethobenzamide), dosage calculation for
    for capsules, 63, 63*f*, 66, 66*f*, 145, 145*f*
    for injection, 73*f*, 74, 137, 137*f*
Time
    in intravenous drug administration, 98–104
    weight and, in dosage calculation, 117–134, 129*f*–134*f*
Time of administration, identification of, in medication orders, 52–53
Titration, and dosage, 117–118, 126–128
Tolbutamide (Orinase), dosage calculation for, 81, 81*f*
Tolinase (tolazamide), dosage calculation for, 65, 65*f*
Trade name, on drug labels, 61
Triazolam (Halcion), dosage calculation for, 63*f*, 63–64, 140, 140*f*
Trimethobenzamide (Tigan). *See* Tigan (trimethobenzamide)
Tubing, for intravenous drug administration, 104, 105*f*
Two-factor medication problems, 85–115, 148*f*–149*f*, 148–152, 202

    for intermittent infusion, and reconstitution, 111–116
    for intravenous medications, drop factors in, 104–110
    for intravenous pumps, 98–104
    for reconstitution, weight and, 93–98
    using quantity and weight, 85–92, 90*f*–93*f*

U

Unit path
    definition of, 38, 202
    in dimensional analysis, 40–41
        in one-factor problems, 53–60

V

Vitamin B12, dosage calculation for, 66, 66*f*
Volume, and dosage, 28–32

W

Wanted quantity
    definition of, 38, 202
    in dimensional analysis, 39–49
        drug label problems using, 62–66
        medication administration problems using, 68–84
        one-factor problems using, 53–60
    in dosage calculation, using weight and time, 117–134, 129*f*–134*f*
    in dosage calculations, using weight, 85–92
    in drop factors, 104–110
    for intravenous medications, 98–104
    for reconstitution, 93–98
    in intermittent infusion, 111–116
Weight
    and dosage, 28–32, 85–92, 90*f*–93*f*
        for children, 117–123
    and reconstitution, 93–98, 94*f*–95*f*, 97*f*

Weight (*continued*)
    time and, in dosage calculation, 117–134, 129*f*–134*f*
    and titration of intravenous medication dose, 117–118, 126–128

X

Xanax (alprazolam), dosage calculation for, 65, 65*f*, 139, 139*f*

Y

Yield, in reconstitution, 93, 96, 168, 202

Z

Zaroxolyn (Metolazone), dosage calculation for, 84–85, 85*f*